The group approach in
nursing practice

The group approach in nursing practice

Gwen D. Marram, R.N., B.S., M.S., Ph.D.

Assistant Superintendent of Nursing Service,
Neuropsychiatric Institute, University of California,
Los Angeles, California

SECOND EDITION

The C. V. Mosby Company

Saint Louis   1978

SECOND EDITION

Copyright © 1978 by The C. V. Mosby Company

Previous edition copyrighted 1973

Printed in the United States of America

Distributed in Great Britain by Henry Kimpton, London

The C. V. Mosby Company
11830 Westline Industrial Drive, St. Louis, Missouri 63141

Library of Congress Cataloging in Publication Data

Marram, Gwen D   1942-
    The group approach in nursing practice.

    Includes bibliographies and index.
    1. Psychiatric nursing.   2.   Group psychotherapy.
I. Title.   [DNLM: 1.   Psychotherapy, Group—Nursing
texts.   2.   Psychiatric nursing.   3.   Nursing, Team.
WY160 M358g]
RC440.M265   1978   616.8'915   77-14584
ISBN   0-8016-3126-2

GW/M/M   9   8   7   6   5   4   3   2   1

To

MERLE
LANCE JOHN
LISA * ALBERT
WILLIAM ALBERT-JOHN
JOANNE

Preface

Groups are ubiquitous and inevitable. They are capable of producing effects of the utmost importance to individuals. The problem for nursing is one of developing an understanding of groups and group work so that desirable consequences for group members can be deliberately enhanced.

It has repeatedly come to my attention, and to the attention of my colleagues in psychiatric–mental health nursing, that a text which treats the scope and nature of group work in nursing is of vital importance to nurses in general and to psychiatric–mental health nurses in particular. Unfortunately, such a text is not available.

The Group Approach in Nursing Practice is designed to fill this gap and to contribute to an understanding of groups and group work with various group members, psychiatric and nonpsychiatric patients, or clients. More specifically, the text describes the potential scope of group work in nursing, illustrates the use of theoretical frameworks in guiding the study and practice of group work, details the steps in establishing, maintaining, and terminating a group, identifies common objectives of the therapist or leader for all group work, and presents a series of group studies that serve to illustrate the implementation of meaningful therapeutic interventions by the nurse in light of various theoretical orientations. In addition the text discusses the therapeutic value of groups that heretofore have not been appreciated for their therapeutic benefits, such as the reference group.

The Group Approach in Nursing Practice is intended to benefit a rather broad audience in nursing, from advanced students and clinicians in psychiatric–mental health nursing to predominately nonpsychiatrically oriented nurse clinicians in general hospitals, clinics, and community health facilities. The book, together with opportunities to engage in supervised group work, will enhance the development of nurse group therapists and nurse group leaders. In addition, it will deepen one's understanding and knowledge of the body of theory about group process, group leadership, and group methods, as well as broaden one's view about the therapeutic potential of groups.

The intended use of groups in clinical practice and in psychiatry-community mental health is perhaps the most promising and exciting innovation of the last three decades. In part this innovation is the direct result of the acknowledgment that groups do exist, that they must be considered to adequately account for human behavior, and that desirable consequences for individuals in groups can be deliberately enhanced. Groups, as it will be explained, offer a number of advantages to their members. These include support, increased problem-solving ability, and, for the psychiatric patient, improved reality testing. No better opportunity exists than in a group experience for individuals to learn how they are uniquely different, yet at the same time, like others. This knowledge is comforting to individuals who view their environment as hostile, foreign, and discouragingly defeating to their aspirations; at the same time this knowledge increases their ability to understand themselves and others. Increased understanding and sensitivity toward others, as well as self-actualization, is the aim of many groups whose members are not concerned with illness or maladjustment, per se, but who wish to further their growth and improve their interpersonal relationships. Groups, then, offer a number of advantages or benefits appropriate for many different types of individuals with many different types of problems and concerns.

It is no longer a question of whether nurses can and should lead groups. The issue is more one of what kind of group work do they do and what unique contribution can they make. This text, because it addresses different kinds of groups, broadens the perspective of nurses as to the potential role they can play in a variety of group modalities.

The presentation of theoretical constructs, which I feel suits the nursing process and role of the nurse group leader, clarifies for the reader how nurses may lead groups differently but complementary to interdisciplinary team members.

The beginning practitioner may be learning group work for the first time. As first-level practitioners, basic nursing students come in contact with a variety of patient constellations who could benefit from group experience. They are learning, or already have learned, preliminary group process, nursing process, and leadership skills. In some instances they have chosen group work as a focus of course work in an area of specialization. These beginning practitioners will find this text invaluable in learning the role of the nurse in mental health, how to integrate theoretical principles with actual practice, and especially what is the role of nurse leader and co-leader in a group.

The advanced practitioner, one experienced in nursing process and the role of the mental health specialist, such as the graduate student in mental health nursing, will find the text helpful as an introduction to a theoretical framework for nurse-led groups in designing a group and coleading, in documenting member change, and in utilizing special techniques to enhance group process and individual members' growth.

This second edition of *The Group Approach in Nursing Practice* reflects important changes and additions. Throughout the text more clinical examples have been used to illustrate the various concepts. The expanding role of nurses in mental health who establish, maintain, and terminate a group of their own design is addressed in particular in an entirely new Chapter 9. The overview of theoretical frameworks pertinent to group work (Chapter 6) includes a new section, "The Behavioral Modification Framework," an important dimension to consider in nurse-led children's groups.

An eclectic theoretical basis for nursing group practice is further reinforced in both Chapters 8 and 9, where nurse leadership functions are defined. The addition of a new case study in Chapter 10 adds to the nurse's knowledge of how to integrate theory and practice, but also illustrates the difficulties and needs of nurses in documenting member behavior change through empirical research.

In summary, it is hoped that the following chapters will enhance nurses' abilities to function effectively as group leaders, group therapists, or cotherapists in the kind of group work suited to them, and that their increased understanding of groups and group work will further their ability to deliberately enhance desirable consequences for individuals in their groups. The first part of the text will examine the scope of group work and the types of groups and their particular objectives, as well as some indications for nurses operating in these groups. The second part will outline the various theoretical frameworks that may guide the nurse's interpretations and interventions. Common objectives of nurses for all group work and application of theory to practice situations will be taken up in the third part of the text. Special considerations for the advanced practitioner coleading, group members' roles, and special techniques are the focus of the fourth and final part of the text.

The ideas and inspiration expressed in this text are the product of encouragement and assistance of many. To Ellie White, although she will never understand the impact of her words, I wish to extend my appreciation as a colleague interested in the right of the nurse specialist to take responsibility for the condition of the group work modality.

I would also like to extend my appreciation to my teachers, students, supervisors, and colleagues in the educational institutions and service agencies in which I have learned, taught, and experienced the group approach.

Special thanks goes to my family whose membership has changed, but whose clear support is what makes things work. To the group members I've touched—members whose names I don't always remember but whose impact has contributed to the growth of so many—I am indebted.

Gwen D. Marram

Contents

PART FOUR

Considerations for the advanced practitioner

The group approach in
nursing practice

Introduction

Building and maintaining an optimum level of mental health is perhaps the health profession's most troublesome task, since such a task requires resources and manpower at every stage of intervention, including the preventive, treatment, and rehabilitative or restorative phases of the health-illness continuum. Unfortunately these resources and manpower are sadly lacking.

In the past, resources were largely confined to the treatment phase. The mental health disciplines for the most part lacked a technology to adequately maintain an optimum level of mental health. The most recent attempts to perform this task are observable in the movement toward community psychiatry and community mental health. The mental health disciplines in general, however, have had a history of meeting needs through the use of somewhat individualistic and idiosyncratic methods. In part, such an approach is the result of a lack of knowledge about the etiology and treatment of psychiatric and psychosocial illness and the confirming findings that individuals are different enough so that certainty of outcome of therapy is still strongly influenced by chance: "What works with one patient, may not work with another." The one-to-one therapeutic relationship appeared to be the best overall method to ensure some therapeutic success, at least with respect to the treatment phase, and thus for some time dominated the psychiatric scene. Adelson[1] noted that the one-to-one relationship approach is still an essential ingredient in various psychiatric–mental health educational programs throughout the country, for both psychiatrists and psychiatric nurses. I might add, however, that in most programs one-to-one relationship therapy is not so much taught with the idea that students will confine their practice following graduation to one-to-one therapy, but with the idea that it provides students with an intensive exposure to diagnostic and treatment problems of one individual patient, an experience that may be generalized to other patient situations. With some exceptions, it has evolved in importance from being the most essential therapeutic tool in the treatment of patients to a respected means of teaching future practitioners who for the most part will be utilizing an array of approaches to patients' and clients' problems, including group psychotherapy, family group therapy, therapeutic community, and modifications of individual relationship therapy, for example, crisis intervention.

In addition to the problems of a lack of manpower and of an effective technology to meet the current demands for prevention, treatment, and rehabilitation or restoration, health professionals face the problem of altering their time perspective and conception of who and what warrant attention.

1

Whittington[2] points out that in a message to the Congress of the United States on February 5, 1963, the late President John F. Kennedy indicated that psychiatry must accept a new emphasis in patient care—that of "quick" treatment of patients in their communities. Prolonged or permanent confinement in institutions that facilitated the use of long-term one-to-one relationship therapy was ideally, if not in actuality, to become obsolete. Although "quick" treatment is not altogether foreign to psychiatry, it does present a difficult dilemma. Long-term one-to-one approaches do not fit this new image; neither, however, does a series of "quick" one-to-one relationships, the feared consequences of abandonment of the long-term one-to-one approach.

The second necessary change in mental health professionals' conceptions of their task includes an expansion of the idea of who the client is and what needs attention. More specifically, with the advent of community mental health it is evident that the individual is only a small part of the picture. Mental health professionals must concern themselves with families, groups, and communities. The unit of analysis and of "treatment," then, can no longer be defined as the individual and his particular personality structure. Families, groups, and communities are the targets of concern. Likewise, with community mental health's emphasis on growth and human potential, as well as on illness per se, persons who did not formerly qualify for attention now are the concern of various mental health professionals and agencies. Thus psychiatry, psychology, and social work have infiltrated the general hospital, the clinics, industry, and business to prevent, treat, and restore to a population heretofore not recognized, optimum psychological growth and mental health.

The problems of building and maintaining an optimum level of mental health and assuring growth are not the task of the core of mental health professionals alone. Such health professionals as general practitioners, public or community health nurses, and members of many other occupational groups, including teachers, social workers, and the clergy, contribute to the growth and health of individuals in groups and in the community. Along with the change in perspective about who and what need attention is a necessary flexibility about what agencies and persons can effectively aid in the establishment and maintenance of an optimum level of mental health.

The importance of nurses with reference to this task has taken on new dimensions. Within the psychiatric–mental health field, the status of nurses is being upgraded. Also, in an attempt to provide services to the nonpatient clientele, graduate psychiatric nurses in particular are being asked to use their skills and knowledges in such nonpsychiatric agencies as the general hospital in liaison services or as clinical specialist consultants. In other areas of nursing, for example, in community health and on medical wards, nurses are expected to assume a more crucial role in the patient's adaptation and adjustment to hospitalization, to illness, and to his community. These trends are concomitant with the increased utilization of a number of allied professionals across various disciplines.

Providing increased manpower through the utilization and recognition of multiple disciplines and occupational groups is not enough. The technology must fit the task. There is no single solution nor approach adequate to ensure mental health; future progress toward such a goal probably depends on several approaches to the problem—one of which is the group approach, which occupies a prominent position in today's health care program. The current and potential scope of group work suggests that a group approach is more than a mere supplement to the one-to-one approach in psychiatry. It is an important and pervasive adjunct throughout the phases of prevention, treatment, and rehabilitation and includes many nonprofessional attempts to alter psychosocial problems as well. In most respects it is an approach well suited to current needs and demands. It tends to be a more efficient approach. More individuals receive attention by fewer professionals, often for shorter periods. Far more important, however, the group approach tends to be an effective means of meeting an array of needs and problems. In addition, groups can offer a number of advantages to persons that other approaches cannot.

Nowhere has it been scientifically documented that patients or clients need to be attended to one-at-a-time, exclusively, in order that psychosocial problems be alleviated, controlled, or prevented. In psychiatry it was believed for some time that certain patients, namely the withdrawn, aggressive, or bizarre, must be treated on an individual basis, at least in the beginning stages of treatment. In nursing in general it was felt that relating to the patient on an individual basis, that is, through individual interviews, was the best way to help him combat his anxieties about hospitalization and illness. What these beliefs fail to appreciate, however, is the fact that these patients are, as are all individuals, operating within the context of some group —informally structured as it may be—on the respective wards or in the community at large. However therapeutic or planned such group experience is, it is affecting their behavior. The problem here becomes one of how best to put this group experience to work for the growth and health of these individuals. In community mental health in particular it is no longer the case that a segment of the patient population cannot benefit from some form of group experience. With the current progress in the use of drugs to control severe psychotic reactions, more and more patients are able to benefit from a planned group experience, whether it takes the form of recreational therapy, a remotivation group experience, or another form. On wards in general hospitals it is becoming more and more clear to nurses that grouping patients together and conducting discussions, for instance, about their illness, is of great importance to the patients' adjustment to their illness, to learn about their problems, and for transition back to the community.

Just as there is no evidence that attending to patients one-at-a-time is the more effective approach, there is much evidence to suggest that patients, clients, and group members in general do benefit from supervised group involvement. Individuals learn about themselves—how they are different and how they are similar to other members in the group. The knowledge that others share the same fears or problems, or have more troubles, seems to be supportive to individuals. For psychiatric patients it serves as an important basis for reality testing. Interestingly enough, group experiences tend to check a delusion or illusion of many persons that they are the only ones who suffer, which for some individuals connotes that they are special or that the whole world is against them. The importance of a group where persons share common problems is borne out in the success of many self-help groups as well. These groups are homogeneous with respect to some problem, for example, drug abuse or alcoholism; they have an impact on their members and a rate of success that no other single therapy can duplicate.

There are more people to react to in various capacities in a group. Catharsis and working through of more problems are enhanced. Characteristically, various roles are taken by persons in groups. Members react not only to the presence of other personalities in the group but also to the roles and positions these persons occupy. A phenomenon of much interest is that persons will often react to the leaders, or therapists if they are psychiatric patients, as parent figures and to group members as siblings. The opportunity to work through such reactions as dependence—reactions that typify earlier relations with important others—can be both helpful and informative to group members, whether they are patients attempting to gain greater insight into their pathology or whether they are individuals merely concerned with improving their interpersonal relationships on the job.

REFERENCES
1. Adelson, D.: A concept of comprehensive community mental health, paper presented at Work Conference in Graduate Education in Psychiatric-Mental Health Nursing, April 24, 1967, University of Maryland.
2. Whittington, H. D.: A third psychiatric revolution—really? Community Ment. Health J. **1:**73, 1965.

PART ONE

The scope of group work

A group approach is appropriate for many individuals with many types of problems and in many different settings. In one sense the group approach has no perceivable boundaries within the framework of prevention, treatment, and restoration and with regard to growth and self-actualization. In psychiatric settings there are various inpatient group psychotherapy groups, outpatient groups, special problem groups, family group therapy groups, and married couples groups that are distinguishable in emphasis. Therapeutic groups, which differ from group psychotherapy groups in that they focus on individuals who are not psychiatric patients and that they have less to do with the treatment of psychiatric illness, can be found in many general hospitals, clinics, nursing homes, industry and business schools, and penal institutions. Self-help groups are increasing in numbers and in kind in the community; these groups resemble therapeutic groups but differ in one important attribute: they are led by the group members themselves.

Some of these groups represent new dimensions in group work; others have been utilized for some time. Each, however, addresses itself to a particular objective such as reeducation, support, or remotivation of the group member.

CHAPTER 1

Group psychotherapy

Introduction

Group psychotherapy, as opposed to therapeutic groups and other group work, is a branch of psychiatry and psychotherapy. It is concerned with the use of the group method and group process as a treatment of psychopathology of persons in the group. Since its beginnings in the early decades of the century, it has undergone extensive expansion and is now practiced by people from a variety of backgrounds, including psychology, nursing, and social work, as well as psychiatry. Group psychotherapy groups may vary in intensity from analytic group psychotherapy based on a psychoanalytic approach to unconscious content, to group psychotherapy based on communication and interpersonal interpretations of the here and now.

Much importance in the past has been attributed to the role of group psychotherapy as a transition for patients terminating individual therapy and to its role in preparing and aiding the patient discharged from the hospital for group living in the community at large. More recently, however, benefits of group psychotherapy to persons who have been maintained in the community without hospitalization have become apparent.

Most patients who are undergoing or who have undergone psychiatric treatment have experienced some breakdown in interpersonal relationships. This experience often leads to feelings of rejection, unworthiness, isolation, and inadequacy. Group psychotherapy has been effective in helping these individuals establish more successful relationships by encouraging them to relate to other people in the group and to resolve some of their former problems and conflicts. An important by-product of this process is that the patient experiences support and increased feelings of self-worth, as well as increased awareness of the reasons for his troubles. Individuals are expected to identify with group goals for health and are encouraged to test out new and more successful patterns of relating and of adapting to the stress they experience.

As Papanek[10] indicates, all patients experience increased self-esteem from the cohesiveness of the group, provoking feelings of belonging and an opportunity for members to be helpful to one another.

The methods by which these group psychotherapy groups help individuals resolve some of their problems in relating to others and help them take on more successful patterns of adapting may differ from group to group. Group psychotherapy groups, for the most part, can be distinguished by their overall emphasis on (1) personality reconstruction, (2) insight without reconstruction, (3) remotivation, (4) problem solving, (5) reeducation, or (6) support. NOTE: Groups that emphasize remotivation, reeducation, and support are often referred to in the literature as group therapy groups, as opposed to group psychotherapy groups. Often these terms are used interchangeably to refer to the same classification of groups. Note the use of the term therapeutic groups in Chapter 2, indicating a third differentiation; this term should not be confused with group therapy. (See Armstrong and Rouslin.[1])

The emphasis of a particular group is dependent on the skills and interests of the therapist, his specific treatment aims for the patients, and the strengths and limitations of the patients composing the group, as well as on the particular treatment philosophy of the agency in which the group is to be conducted. Quite often, however, to adequately account for patients' needs a single group may shift in emphasis, for example, from support to insight, or may have a dual emphasis such as support and problem solving throughout all its sessions.

Group psychotherapy groups include a number of inpatient and outpatient or clinic groups with one—and in some instances, more than one—of the above emphases. In addition to this system of classification, however, there are categories that further differentiate the aims of group psychotherapy experience for patients. Such categories may refer to the context in which the group operates and to its focus. Group psychotherapy in a therapeutic milieu, for example, is part of an entire program to provide a ward culture that fosters healthy personalities. Family group therapy groups, as well as married couples' groups, extend the focus of group treatment from the patients to those persons who are affected by and who affect the patient, with the idea that family members are a part of the psychopathological system that resulted in the client becoming the identified patient. Special problem groups serve to specify the focus with reference to the problem area of the patient, such as adolescent adjustment, alcoholism, or narcotic addiction. NOTE: Groups that prepare patients for discharge and that orient them to the hospital setting are not taken up as forms of group psychotherapy. This is essentially because such groups have much potential in a variety of settings other than the psychiatric hospital and because adaptation to a new, strange, and sometimes frightening environment is viewed as a phenomenon not necessarily bound to psychiatric explanation and therefore somewhat inappropriate to psychiatric treatment or intervention alone.

The selection of patients or clients for a particular type of group therapeutic experience must take into consideration the various emphases and foci described above. There are, however, some general guidelines that may direct the selection of patients for group psychotherapy groups. Basically, one must consider the needs of the patients and the objectives of group psychotherapy to ascertain whether this group experience will play an important role in the patient's treatment program. Secondly, one must determine whether the patients will be able to participate without seriously interfering with the realization of treatment benefits of the group for other members. Such decisions may be based on (1) the nature and status of the patient's illness, (2) his potential strengths in interpersonal relationships, and (3) certain similarities or differences between patients that would influence a member's capacity to relate to other members of the group, and they to him.[9]

An additional criterion, and an important one, is the availability of patients. A typical group might contain eight to twelve patients with varying diagnoses. The availability of patients is determined by the natural influx or turnover of patients, but also by the agency and its administrative staff. When a group is confined to a particular ward or unit, the selection of patients is likely to be more restricted. Administrative policies and treatment practices may also restrict the availability of patients, sometimes more so with groups led by nurses. An agency, for example, may have specific ideas about the position nurses should occupy with reference to the administration of therapy. It may specify that the nurse's role should be a cotherapy role and should serve a primarily supportive function, with a select segment of the patient population. In this case nurses may need to negotiate their own role in the agency within these limitations, but in light of their capacity to function with a variety of patients in different types of group psychotherapy groups.

Other criteria for the selection of patients refer to a number of specific personal traits of the patients. These include such factors as age, sex, socioeconomic and cultural background, intelligence, ability to communicate, motivation, the severity of the illness, previous group experience, and aggressiveness. It is important to consider how the particular personal traits of patients will combine or interact in the group. For example, it may be less helpful to patients if the therapist combined highly intelligent and insightful patients with patients extremely limited in regard to intellect and cultural endowment. It would also be unwise to include a fearful, submissive patient in a group of extremely exploitative and aggressive sociopathic patients. This is not to say, however, that all groups should be rigidly homogeneous in all respects. Marked differences among members are often productive and stimulate interaction. In most instances, due to the restricted availability of patients, such rigid homogeneity would be impossible even if it were desirable or necessary. A degree of homogeneity, however, to mediate differences and enhance the formation of cohesiveness in the group so that it will not break into diverse subgroups, is something nurses must be concerned with and something they must strive to achieve in the selection of patients for their group.

Just as nurses may need to achieve a "fit" in the selection of patients for their group, they must be cognizant of how their own personal attributes combine with those of the patients in their group. Their specific leadership skills and knowledge of group dynamics and psychopathology are extremely important; but just as critical is their tolerance for specific behaviors in a group setting. Some nurses, for example, may be more skillful with articulate patients who are capable of developing insight into their problems through the group experience. Still other nurses may be better able to tolerate regression in patients and would be more useful in chronic psychotic patient groups, groups that have goals of supporting and remotivating patients.

Inpatient groups

Within psychiatric institutions are a number of group psychotherapy groups that vary in intensity and are distinguishable in aim. The aim and intensity of these groups depends on the philosophy and treatment practices of the particular ward and staff as well as on the capacities of the patient and the nature of his illness. The aim or emphasis of these groups ranges from being personality reconstruction oriented to offering support. (For further description of groups that are personality reconstruction, insight, and support oriented, see Wolberg.[15])

Therapists such as Leopold[7] suggest that group psychotherapy for inpatients differs from that for outpatients. Inpatient groups must be aligned with the total treatment program. Usually there is a series of interrelated group activities that are most often differentiated from one another by the levels of members' illness.

Personality reconstruction

Groups whose aim it is to achieve personality reconstruction in its patients require an intensive analytic focus on individuals in the group. Analytic group psychotherapy as described by Slavson[12] and others belongs in this category. Such groups may employ dream material and free association along with individual interviews in the group setting. Essentially each individual is analyzed within a group context. Because a number of problems are covered by this type of group, the benefits of increased catharsis are operant. The interpersonal problems between members are also worked through, but with a decided focus on the roots of these problems originating in the patients' former relationships. Patients in these groups are expected to modify their behavior patterns and in some instances to abandon former defensive mechanisms.

Insight without reconstruction

A less intensive type of group therapy and one that focuses more on the here and now are groups that aim to provide increased insight but that do not attempt major personality reconstruction. Such groups are more widely used in a variety of psychiatric settings than are reconstruction groups, perhaps because of the greater emphasis on interpersonal and communication theories in psychiatry—theories that are less concerned with the unconscious. These groups are also useful and appropriate to a greater variety of patients. The focus of the group for the most part includes the interpersonal problems of patients in the here and now in the group—problems between patients and family, between patients and staff, and among patients on the ward—through an analysis of members' communication and interaction with others. These groups tend to differ from problem-solving groups per se. The exploration of problems in the insight group is usually of greater depth, and in some cases solutions are not the chief concern, but rather an emotional integration and intellectual insight that increases the patients' understanding of the problem and that makes prior behavior (usually that which is involved in the problematic situation) unnecessary. In general, insight groups attempt to provide group members with increased insight about how they affect others and how they are affected by others and with alternative ways of reacting or behaving.

Problem solving

Problem-solving groups concentrate less on in-depth understanding and analysis and more on circumscribed problems of the patient. Such problems may include those related to orientation and discharge but also include more general problems of relating to other patients, to staff, and to the institutional regime. Usually individual problems are isolated for discussion in the group; a patient may describe a concern, for example, how to demonstrate that he is ready for a ward job assignment. Other patients may contribute their ideas and experiences. Some direction for the patient with the problem usually surfaces from such a discussion, and in the following sessions patients may discuss the results of applying the solution to the problem. Problem-solving techniques can be employed by a therapist in almost every kind of group; in problem-solving groups, however, such techniques are central to its operation. These groups are frequently the model utilized by ward and community groups.

Remotivation and reeducation

Other groups that are utilized frequently as models for ward and community groups are groups that strive to remotivate or reeducate or both. Remotivation groups use a variety of techniques to encourage patients to communicate or interact with one another. These techniques often include activity of some kind in which patients may participate together as a group. Some groups use games or sports; others, art work or listening to music. Usually these techniques are a means to motivate patients to interact with each other and are not continued throughout all the sessions. When patients are ready, talking usually replaces activity. These groups are extremely useful with withdrawn patients and with patients who have undergone long-term institutionalization that has produced apathy, isolated detachment, and social impoverishment. Bell[2] and Ward[14] remind us of the difficulties in treating the chronic inpatient when we rely on verbal exchange as a means of establishing relationships in groups. Reeducation groups are also useful for withdrawn, institutionalized patients. These groups attempt to encourage in patients appropriate social and interactional responses. Often the therapist is teaching, by informing and reinforcing certain behaviors, what is the norm or the accepted behavior. Patients who have undergone long-term institutionalization, and in some cases human interactional neglect, are often not attuned to what is appropriate or acceptable. Patients who have suffered chronic and regressive psychiatric illness are also likely to be socially inept and therefore are good candidates for this type of group experience.

Supportive

An emphasis on support, like that on problem solving, may be found in many types of group psychotherapy groups. Such an emphasis, however, may relate only tangentially to the overall intent or long-term objective of the therapist. Depending on the strength of the patients in the group at any one time, the therapist may choose to reinforce defensive reactions rather than to push for personality reconstruction, insight, problem solving, reeducation, or any combination of these. Groups whose main intent is to reinforce existing defenses of patients may be referred to as supportive therapy groups. This type of group, then, does not seek insight or personality reconstruction but helps patients maintain a functional or semifunctional adaptation to their environment, given the defense system of the patient. These groups benefit many patients, both chronically and acutely ill, who are perceived to have weak egos or to be unable to cope with revelation of fears and conflicts but who need reassurance from social relations and interpersonal contact to maintain their current level of reality testing. The focus is on the here and now situations of the patients, for example, on common interests and concerns about ward living. The therapist does not threaten defenses used by the patients in the group. He is concerned that anxiety of patients be kept at a minimum so they can tolerate the presence of others in the group and the group setting itself.

Nurses in the psychiatric–mental health setting are most frequently involved with groups that are supportive, problem solving, reeducation, or remotivation oriented, and to a lesser degree, with insight groups. Nurses are not widely involved in leading reconstruction groups. This is probably for two essential reasons: (1) reconstruction or analytically oriented groups are utilized less frequently in the majority of psychiatric settings, and (2) the current status of nurses' skills and knowledges dictates how such groups will operate. Unfortunately few nurses are equipped to lead analytic groups, even if they were acknowledged as capable of operating in such a capacity.

Nurses have for some time participated in group interaction that lends support, remotivates, reeducates, or aids patients in problem solving, often in their minute-to-minute interactions with small informal groups on the ward. That they should lead formal groups based on one or more of these aims is understandable. Increasingly their ability for operating in a capacity to further patients' insights has been both developed and recognized. It is not unusual to find nurses coleading such groups with psychiatrists, psychologists, and psychiatric social workers, and even with other nurses. Current preparation in psychiatric–mental health graduate nursing programs is aimed at developing nurse–therapists to operate alone as sole therapist or with another nurse as a cotherapist in insight groups.

The necessary preparation for nurses who wish to lead group psychotherapy groups varies with the particular emphasis of the group. Basically, however, a knowledge of psychotherapy and psychopathology, of group dynamics, and of the benefits of groups is important to working in any psychotherapy group. They will need, in addition, group leadership skills and an ability to employ various psychotherapeutic techniques. Insight groups require nurses to have, in addition to these skills and knowledges, insight into their own behavior toward individuals in the group, a keen sense of timing with reference to interventions, and a capacity to judge patients' reactions to and tolerance of self-realization and self-revelation. An ability to conceptualize, to analyze, and to empathize with patients achieving increased insight is important if patients are to feel confident with their leadership. A theoretical background that draws on analytic, interpersonal, and communication frameworks will be useful in guiding interventions and suggesting interpretations. Supervision of their experiences by an objective and experienced staff member is helpful and advisable.

In supportive, problem-solving, and remotivation-reeducation groups, the special techniques of increasing patients' self-esteem, employing problem-solving processes, stimulating patient interaction, and reinforcing appropriate behavior, respectively, will be useful to nurses in making meaningful therapeutic interventions with regard to the particular aim of the group. Theoretical frameworks, for example, those from social psychology, psychology and human behavior, and from education, will provide a basis for many of their interventions.

Inpatient milieu—the therapeutic community

It must be remembered that within various psychiatric–mental health settings there are always overlapping and interacting group influences that can affect patients. Not only are patients exposed to structured groups but also to multiple informal interactions with groups on the ward. Staff interact with patients in a number of formal and informal meetings.

The recognition that patients' therapeutic experiences are not, nor need be, solely the result of organized and insulated group efforts at scheduled periods of the day has done much to alter conceptions of what happens in the minute-to-minute interaction of patients and between patients and staff. Prior to this recognition such interaction was viewed as slightly less significant and somewhat less valid than the more formal meetings, however reliable a measure it was of a patient's current emotional state. Nor was this interaction appreciated for its capacity to affect patients' behavior. Nurses, perhaps because of their continual exposure to such interaction, were probably the only group cognizant of the diagnostic and therapeutic potential of this interaction.

Psychiatric wards that are considered continuously functioning therapeutic milieus are therapeutic communities. The therapeutic community, based on group principles, represents as much a philosophy of treatment as it does a type of approach. The idea of a therapeutic community began to seriously permeate the psychiatric orientation of wards after World War II. Initially it seemed to take hold in Western Europe where there was a shortage of therapists and a great sense of community responsibility.[6]

There are several operational components of the therapeutic community approach. These include extensive use of occupational, recreational, and industrial therapy programs, vocational rehabilitation, development of patient government, group psychotherapy groups, and group works. Some outcomes of employing the therapeutic community approach have resulted in what Roberts[11] and others have identified as open wards. Open wards afford greater control to patients, for example, over their possessions, greater opportunities for communication between patients and staff and among patients, and increased opportunities for patient activity.

It is the responsibility of nurses in a therapeutic community to help create and maintain a culture that may foster healthy personalities. They are expected to support and encourage the patients in every phase of their treatment and in their minute-to-minute interaction with patients and to convey appropriate responses and behavior. Such norms, transmitted to patients by way of the nurses, are part of the total therapeutic community culture, and in some instances are norms the patient would be obliged to abide by in the extrahospital community. Nurses encourage the patients to examine their interactions within the community setting. In the overall therapeutic community regime, as Zalba and Abels[17] suggest, nurses must intervene in a variety of ways in the group life of patients; that is, through spontaneous as well as planned instruction for the group by directly "rescuing" members in difficulty and by confronting individuals and groups with their actual behavior.

The success and benefits of the therapeutic community seem to arise in part from the fact that patients and staff are interacting in a closely integrated community group. Such integration and its benefits are noted by Roberts[11] in his experiences with the therapeutic approach in a state hospital in Wisconsin. Because of the cohesion of the group, members gain a sense of personal responsibility and self-respect. These outcomes are also shared by staff members. In this cohesive community, group controls are used to diminish bizarre behavior of individuals while encouraging more socially acceptable and desirable behavior. As Roberts noted, the disruptive social interaction patterns of members are frequently abandoned when they as persons are accepted by the group.

Within the closely integrated therapeutic community, patients' behavior is observed, scrutinized, examined, and discussed by all the members of the community. Patients learn about their own problems as well as about those of other patients. Such experiences, then, as Maxwell Jones[5] noted of his treatment of a group of sociopaths, afford increased insight and the possibility of better control over one's behavior.

Outpatient and clinic groups

The small group in the protected environment of a clinic is an important means for continuing to help the mental patient toward recovery after his discharge from the hospital. The continued contact with therapeutic agents and with people who are also recovering enables him to gain support for his incorporation into the community at large and for building on his insight about himself in interpersonal relationships.

Although many outpatient or clinic groups are part of an overall aftercare program for discharged patients, they are also utilized for individuals who have never been hospitalized but who need the cloister of the group situation to maintain or enhance a particular level of psychosocial adaptation to their community, their job, family, and everyday life experiences. The aim or emphasis of these groups is frequently one of increasing insight and problem-solving ability as well as support. Although outpatient groups do reflect the general array of emphases found in the inpatient setting, they are often less likely to include remotivation groups, yet more likely to include analytic groups. Their aim, as in the inpatient setting, is determined by the purpose and philosophy of the agency, the needs of the clients, and the training and philosophy of the staff.

In addition to the wide variety of outpatient groups that operate in public or private psychiatric agencies, a number of such groups are conducted in the community at large and often involve many nonpsychiatric personnel. These groups may operate in settings such as halfway houses and day-care centers. It is believed that they ease the adaptation of patients to the community, continue the process of adjustment begun in the hospital, and lessen the number of relapses.

As was noted above, outpatient and clinic groups may differ little from inpatient groups in their aim or emphasis, which may range from personality reconstruction to a supportive orientation. But they also may focus on a special problem or may include persons affected by and who affect the patient. For the most part, outpatient and clinic groups represent a continuation of the types of groups found in a hospital setting.

There are certain ways, however, in which these groups differ from inpatient groups. These differences are a result of various factors related to the patients' being in the community and not in a hospital environment. Persons in the community or discharged to the community are often more in contact with reality and have achieved a higher level of psychosocial adaptation. Surveillance of group members by the therapist is limited to the periodic group contacts for the most part. And persons in the community are involving family members in their pathological syndromes or are suffering increased strain in the readjustment to a family group system of interaction. These factors are accommodated for through several structural differences in the group other than the group's particularized aim: (1) meetings may be held less frequently—once weekly versus daily or two to three times weekly in the inpatient setting; (2) some part of the meetings may be focused on the individuals to ascertain their current progress; in some cases outpatient groups are not accompanied by individual surveillance, and the therapist may feel the need to check on the individual's well-being through individual interview techniques within the group setting; and (3) groups may more often involve the patient's family—his children, or spouse, or all of them—for one or more sessions or as the basis of the group, for example, in family group therapy or married couples groups.

Nurses' roles in outpatient and clinic groups resemble those in the inpatient setting. They may be expected to colead or in some cases to be the sole leader of these groups. In mental health centers and many outpatient departments, as recognized members of the treatment team, nurses increasingly have an equal responsibility in leading therapy groups. The skills and knowledges required to operate in the outpatient groups are similar to those needed in the inpatient setting. There are some important differences, however. Nurses do not have the advantage of extensive observation of the patients or clients that they would have if these individuals were hospitalized. Their observation skills and ability to synthesize information derived from infrequent contacts with patients must be well developed. In cases where a crisis intervention orientation governs the operation of the agency, they must also be able to make every intervention profitable with regard to the patients' well-being.

One of the foremost problems in leading outpatient or aftercare groups is the fact that the leader cannot always control attendance, at least to the extent possible in an inpatient setting. Much has been written about this problem. Basically an outpatient group is not a "captive" audience—it must be captured. Lyon[8] refers to the problem of establishing trust in these groups when attendance is sporadic, and therefore cohesion and trust are haphazardly established. The very fact that the leader cannot control attendance—that members resist through absences—renders him impotent. Spratlen[13] emphasizes the need to pay attention to the lifestyles and cultures of the patient population in order to become more creditable to the patient in the community. Contracts with members promising attendance and phone-call follow-up are additional strategies the nurse leader of an outpatient group should consider.

Special-problem groups

The range of group therapy groups that focus on special problems is extensive. Such groups can be found in both inpatient and outpatient facilities and increasingly in such agencies as centers for special problems. Basically they elicit homogeneity for the purpose of attacking directly a problem of concern to all the patients or clients in the group. Such groups include adolescent group therapy groups, group therapy with alcoholics, group therapy with narcotic addicts, and group therapy with the sexually maladjusted. Homogeneity in these groups is thought to be a powerful influence on such problems and may best create a climate of acceptance and encourage serious discussion of one's fears and concerns. Beginning research on problems of addiction and alcoholism seem to indicate that homogeneous grouping of these persons is far more successful than mixing them in heterogeneous group therapy groups. Homogeneous groups are able to penetrate more quickly the defenses of addicts and alcoholics, defenses that perpetuate excuses to drink and to take drugs. In many instances, special problem groups are dealing with socially disapproved of behaviors. When patients or clients who exhibit socially disapproved of behaviors are put together in a group, they experience a greater feeling of being understood and accepted; whereas in heterogeneous groups they anticipate discrimination and social isolation, reactions that may in fact occur.

Preparation of nurses to lead special problem groups is enhanced by specific skill and knowledge related to the problem area. For example, group therapy with alcoholics requires specific knowledge of the alcoholic personality, the dynamics of his adaptation and adjustment to life problems, and a knowledge of his resistance to treatment. Nurses need to know what techniques work best in helping him choose and adjust to alternative patterns of behavior. With respect to drug addicts, they will want to be equipped with an array of confrontation techniques. Such techniques are utilized by a number of Synanon groups and prove to be quite helpful in the treatment of addicts. Special-problem groups with adolescents require in-depth knowledge of human development and the social, emotional, and physical problems of adolescence.

In their work with special-problem groups, nurses will need to keep in mind that the special problem that brings the client to the agency for treatment is a symptom and not the illness itself. Therefore, although they are attempting to modify or eliminate the symptom or problem, they must be aware of the underlying psychosocial phenomenon that causes the client to exhibit the problem in the first place. The degree to which therapists deal with the underlying cause, more than with the symptom, will depend on the emphasis of the group, the individual therapists' skill and knowledge, and the philosophy of the agency under whose aegis the therapy is conducted.

Family, multiple family, and married couples groups

Family group therapy and multiple family group therapy groups are also employed both on an inpatient and on an outpatient basis. Essentially the aim of both groups is to improve interaction between the patient and his family members; generally the major focus is on the nuclear family, that is, the patient's mother, father, and siblings if the patient is a child. (Recent attention has been given the establishment of intergenerational groups such as with grandparents, parents, and children of the same sex. Mother and daughter groups and siblings and patient groups represent innovative combinations of family and group therapy.) The family may be treated as a group of individuals, with one member being the "identified patient" in the group. The family itself, however, and its interactional processes are considered pathological.

Family group therapy and multiple family group therapy groups resemble family therapy per se.

Family therapy is a form of psychotherapy that treats all family members by seeing the group in conjoint sessions. The sessions focus not on the individual who is identified as the patient, but on the total family. (See Handleman.[4]) Both family therapy and family group therapy, terms often used interchangeably in the literature, are based on the idea that within the family system is the dysfunction that produced the symptoms of the identified patient. Therefore the therapist needs to see the family members together in a group to get a clearer picture of what goes on within the family. Some therapists argue, however, that family therapy is different from family group therapy in important ways. Family therapy, it is suggested, uses principles and techniques of group psychotherapy to less an extent than might be expected. The therapist in family therapy as Boszormenyi[3] notes is involved in family members' existence in a far more global manner. Also, family groups, unlike other group therapy groups, are composed of persons who have had a history of adaptation to one another with special bonds of relationship and familiarity. The family therapist establishes a relationship with the family, which is an interpersonal *organization* having an established history and prospects of a continued future together.[16] There is much feeling among some family therapists that the distinctive features of family therapy are obscured if it is regarded as a form of group therapy. Still other therapists prefer to view the family with regard to small group behavior; these therapists will often use the term family group therapy when discussing or describing the family therapy approach.

The combined family approach or multiple family group therapy may be viewed as one variation of family group therapy. Multiple family group therapy groups consist of a number of families (usually not more than four or five, but depending on the size of the families) seen simultaneously in a group. Included in this group are the identified patients of each individual family. The combined family approach has the added advantage of increasing families' insights into their own and other families' problems. Families are able to compare and constrast their own interactional patterns with those of other families. This experience lends support as well as contributes to a family's knowledge of how they are uniquely different or similar to other families in their communication patterns and interactional networks. Often families will become aware of why they do not have the problems of other families, but also, why other families do not have the problems they themselves exhibit.

An additional variation of the family group therapy approach is the married couples group. These groups include the spouse of the identified patient. Within the framework of family group therapy the therapist may vary the combination of family members to be seen. Some therapists see the children as well as the patient throughout all the sessions, whereas others may not include children at all, or may include them in a few key sessions only. Married couples groups begin with the patient and his (her) spouse; at the discretion of the therapist the children may be brought into the group at a later time, usually for not more than three or four sessions.

Married couples groups may include as many as six or seven couples. In most instances one partner has been identified as a patient. It is not unusual, however, that both husband and wife suffer problems of low self-esteem.

The role of nurses in family group therapy, multiple family group therapy, and married couples groups has been one primarily of a cotherapy relationship with a psychiatric social worker, psychiatrist, or psychologist. More and more, especially in outpatient clinics, nurses are being recognized as capable of leading such groups or of operating as cotherapists with other nurses. The nurses who choose to operate in this capacity will require specific skills and knowledges. In addition to the basic leadership skills—knowledge of psychotherapy and psychopathology and of group dynamics—they will need special skills and knowledges relating to the family and to family therapy. Of the abundant theories related to family therapy and family dynamics, the most renowned are communication theory and conjoint family therapy principles. Some therapists believe that game theory also is helpful in explaining family dynamics. A number of specialized programs in family therapy centers, as well as in graduate nursing programs, focus on preparing nurse-therapists in family therapy and family group therapy. Usually these programs require nurses to have mastered a year of graduate preparation in psychiatric–mental health nursing. This fact is becoming increasingly modified, however, by those programs which believe that first-year graduate nurses can be prepared in beginning skills and knowledges of family therapy and which incorporate family therapy theory and practice in the first year of students' graduate programs.

REFERENCES

1. Armstrong, S. W., and Rouslin, S.: Group psychotherapy in nursing practice, New York, 1963, The Macmillan Co.
2. Bell, R.: Activity as a tool in group therapy, Perspect. Psychiatr. Care **8:**84, 1970.
3. Boszormenyi-Nagy, I.: Intensive family therapy as process. In Boszormenyi-Nagy, I., and Framo, J. L., editors: Intensive family therapy, New York, 1966, Harper & Row, Publishers.

4. Handleman, B. H.: Family therapy. In Kalkman, M.: Psychiatric nursing, ed. 3, New York, 1967, McGraw-Hill Book Co., p. 258.
5. Jones, M.: Social psychiatry, Springfield, Ill., 1962, Charles C Thomas, Publisher, p. 68.
6. Kalkman, M. E.: Psychiatric nursing, ed. 2, New York, 1967, McGraw-Hill Book Co., p. 10.
7. Leopold, H.: Selective group approaches with psychotic patients in hospital settings, Am. J. Psychother. **30:**95-102, 1976.
8. Lyon, G.: Trust in the non-hospitalized group, Perspect. Psychiatr. Care **8:**64-72, 1970.
9. National Association of Social Workers: Use of groups in the psychiatric setting, proceedings of the Workshop Conference on the Group Process in the Psychiatric Setting, sponsored by the National Association of Social Workers in cooperation with the Continuing Education Service and the School of Social Work, Michigan State University, East Lansing, Mich., June 1958, p. 85.
10. Papanek, H.: Therapeutic and antitherapeutic factors in group relations, Am. J. Psychother. **23:**400, 1969.
11. Roberts, L. M.: Group meetings in a therapeutic community. In Benber, H., editor: Therapeutic community, Springfield, Ill., 1959, Charles C Thomas, Publisher, pp. 132-137.
12. Slavson, S. R.: A textbook in analytic group psychotherapy, New York, 1964, International Universities Press.
13. Spratlen, L.: A black client group in day treatment, Perspect. Psychiatr. Care **12:**176-182, 1974.
14. Ward, J.: The sounds of silence: group psychotherapy with non-verbal patients, Perspect. Psychiatr. Care **7:**12, 1974.
15. Wolberg, L. R.: Techniques of psychotherapy, New York, 1964, Grune & Stratton.
16. Wynne, L. C.: Some indications and contraindications for exploratory family therapy. In Boszormenyi-Nagy, I., and Framo, J. L., editors: Intensive family therapy, New York, 1966, Harper & Row, Publishers, p. 305.
17. Zalba, S. R., and Abels, P.: Training the nurse in psychiatric group work, J. Psychiatr. Nurs. Ment. Health Serv. **8:**9, 1970.

SUGGESTED READINGS
Introduction

Armstrong, S. W., and Rouslin, S.: Group psychotherapy in nursing practice, New York, 1963, The Macmillan Co.
Beard, N., and Scott, P.: The efficacy of group therapy by nurses for hospitalized patients, Nurs. Res. **24:**120-124, 1975.
Corsini, R. J.: Methods of group psychotherapy, New York, 1957, McGraw-Hill Book Co.
Hinckley, R., and Hermann, L.: Group treatment in psychotherapy, Minneapolis, 1951, University of Minnesota Press.
Kadis, A., et. al.: A practicum of group psychotherapy, New York, 1963, Harper & Row, Publishers.
Locke, N.: Bibliography on group psychotherapy, New York, 1954, American Group Psychotherapy Association.
Murphy, G.: Group psychotherapy in our society. In Rosenbaum, M., and Berger, M., editors: Group psychotherapy and group function, ed. 2, New York, 1975, Basic Books, Inc., Publishers.
Powermaher, F., and Frank, J.: Group psychotherapy, Cambridge, Mass., 1953, Harvard University Press.
Rosenbaum, M., and Berger, M., editors: Group psychotherapy and group function, ed. 2, New York, 1975, Basic Books, Inc., Publishers.
Sager, C. J.: Discussion: the relationship of group psychotherapy to other group modalities in mental health, Int. J. Group Psychother. **20:**540-544, 1970.

Wolberg, L., and Schwartz, E., editors: Group therapy, New York, 1973, Intercontinental Medical Book Corp.

Yalom, I. C.: The theory and practice of group psychotherapy, ed. 2, New York, 1975, Basic Books, Inc., Publishers.

Inpatient groups

Annesley, P. T.: A rehabilitation unit on group therapy lines for long-stay patients, Psychiatr. Q. **35:**231-235, 1961.

Battegay, R.: Psychotherapy of schizophrenics in small groups, Int. J. Group Psychother. **15:**316-320, 1965.

Horowitz, B., and Weisberg, P.: Techniques for the group psychotherapy of acute psychosis, Int. J. Group Psychother. **16:**42, 1966.

Kelman, H. C.: The role of the group in the induction of therapeutic change, Int. J. Group Psychother. **13:**399-432,1963.

Maurin, J.: Regressed patients in group therapy, Perspect. Psychiatr. Care **8:**131-135, 1970.

Schiff, S. B., and Glassmain, S. M.: Large and small group therapy in a state mental health center, Int. J. Group Psychother. **19:**150-157, 1969.

Stotsky, B. A., and Zolik, E. S.: Group psychotherapy with psychotics: 1921-1963, a review, Int. J. Group Psychother. **15:**321-344, 1965.

Inpatient milieu—the therapeutic community

Dember, H. C., editor: Therapeutic community, Springfield, Ill., 1959, Charles C Thomas, Publisher.

Fidler, J.: The day hospital: a multimodel group therapy. In Wolberg, L., and Aronson, M., editors: Group therapy, 1975: an overview, New York, 1975, Intercontinental Medical Book Corp.

Gardner, K.: Patient groups in a therapeutic community, Am. J. Nurs. **71:**528-531, 1971.

Jones, M.: A passing glance at the therapeutic community in 1964, Int. J. Group Psychother. **15:**5-10, 1965.

Siegel, N.: What is a therapeutic community, Nurs. Outlook **12:**49-51, 1964.

Wax, J.: Analyzing a therapeutic community meeting, Int. J. Group Psychother. **15:**29-36, 1965.

Wilmer, H. A.: Social psychiatry in action: a therapeutic community, Springfield, Ill., 1958, Charles C Thomas, Publisher.

Outpatient and clinic groups

Comstock, B., and Jones, M.: Group therapy as a treatment technique for severely disturbed outpatients, Hosp. Community Psychiatry **26:**677-679, 1975.

Spotnitz, H.: The borderline schizophrenic in group psychotherapy, Int. J. Group Psychother. **7:**155-174, 1957.

Holmes, M., Le Fley, D., and Werner, J.: Creative nursing in day and night care centers, Am. J. Nurs. **62:**86-90, 1962.

Levene, H., Patterson, U., Murphy, B., et. al.: The aftercare of schizophrenics: an evaluation of group and individual approaches, Psychiatr. Q. **44:**296-304, 1970.

Special problem groups

Birk, L., Miller, E., and Cohler, B.: Group psychotherapy for homosexual men by male-female cotherapists. In Sager, C., and Kaplan, H., editors: Progress in group and family therapy, New York, 1972, Brunner/Mazel, pp. 680-759.

Dolan, L.: Intake group in the alcoholism outpatient clinic, J. Stud. Alcohol. **36:**496-499, 1975.

Fox, R.: Group psychotherapy with alcoholics. In Rosenbaum, M., and Berger, M., editors: Group psychotherapy and group function, ed. 2, New York, 1975, Basic Books, Inc., Publishers.

Riess, D.: The suicide six: observations in suicidal behavior and group function, J. Soc. Psychiatry **14:**201-212, 1968.

Family, multiple family, and married couples groups

Bell, J.: Recent advances in family group therapy. In Rosenbaum, M., and Berger, M., editors: Group psychotherapy and group function, ed. 2, New York, 1975, Basic Books, Inc., Publishers.

Benson, L., et. al.: Family communication systems, Small Group Behav. **6:**91-105, 1975.

Bulbulyan, A.: The psychiatric nurse as family therapist, Perspect. Psychiatr. Care **7:**58-67, 1969.

Sager, C., and Kaplan, H. S., editors: Progress in group and family therapy, New York, 1972, Brunner/Mazel, pp. 255-587.

CHAPTER 2

Therapeutic groups

Introduction

Traditionally the use of group psychotherapy techniques has been largely confined to the treatment of the mentally ill. Presently, however, the use of these techniques is more widespread. Group psychotherapy techniques, in the broad sense of the term, are currently employed in counseling a number of client populations, for example, the physically ill, the aged, youths with psychosocial developmental problems, and socially displaced members of the community. As the use of these group techniques broadens, it is helpful to differentiate therapeutic group approaches from the traditional form of group psychotherapy groups. Although the distinction between therapeutic and group therapy groups may seem to be purely an arbitrary one in some instances, there are several important differences worth specifying.

Therapeutic and group therapy groups may be differentiated according to (1) how big a role emotional stress has played in the individual's current level of health (or illness) and (2) the primary or central objective of the group experience. In group psychotherapy groups, members' emotional stress is of paramount concern; the central or primary objective is the treatment of the emotional disturbance manifested in members' thoughts, feelings, and behavior. In therapeutic groups, the classification of group practice to which this chapter is dedicated, emotional stress in most cases is *secondary* to some physical illness, normal growth and developmental crisis, or social maladjustment. In this case the primary objective of the group experience is not treatment, but prevention, education, and, to some extent, crisis orientation.

Where the group is conducted and by whom are sometimes indicative of the differences in the two groups. This is not always the case, however. Presently many mental health professionals are engaged in group work in nonpsychiatric agencies. (Likewise, treatment of psychiatric illness is not their primary objective.) One can also find more and more individuals who are not members of the mental health profession engaged in group work of some kind. The role emotional disturbance plays and the primary objective of the group, then, are far more reliable indicators of these two forms of group practice than simply who leads the group and where the group is conducted.

Therapeutic groups, unlike group psychotherapy groups per se, have developed from a variety of disciplinary efforts, including those of social work, psychology, and nursing, as well as psychiatry. Dr. Joseph Pratt first introduced the idea of therapeutic groups in 1905 when he organized tuberculosis patients together in small groups for a therapeutic purpose. Therapeutic groups in medical hospital settings were utilized in the 1940s in the training and practice of psychiatric social workers. Since then, these groups led by psychologists and social workers began to appear more frequently in general hospitals, in the community with families, in clinics and rehabilitation centers, and in detention homes for delinquent children. Much of this work with groups was referred to as group counseling.

The use of therapeutic groups in nursing practice is probably the result of at least three important factors: (1) nurses' involvement with social workers in groups of this kind, (2) the growing attention of all nurses to the psychosocial factors of illness and growth and development, and (3) the increased interest in mental health nursing in group work with a variety of nonpsychiatric patient populations. The coexistence of social workers and nurses in health and welfare agencies has frequently led to colleagueal relationships despite much opinion otherwise; these relationships have encouraged the use of nurses as coleaders in groups led by social workers and eventually to the leadership of such groups by nurses themselves. Concomitant with this movement has been the increasing interest and concern of nurses —in the schools, in community health, and on medical-surgical wards, for example —for the psychosocial ramifications of growth and development and illness, where the illness originates from a psychological problem or where illness and hospitalization create secondary psychological stress. Paralleling this concern for the mental health of nonpsychiatric clients has been the interest of mental health nurses in these nonpsychiatric clients. Currently students in graduate programs are exploring the various uses of therapeutic groups with a number of these client types, for example, with patients on medical-surgical units, such as kidney transplant, preoperative, cardiac, stroke, cancer, or ulcer patients, with high school and primary school children requiring guidance and counseling, with the aged in nursing homes and convalescent hospitals, and with such clients in the community at large as unwed mothers and delinquent youths.

The focus of therapeutic groups differs essentially in two respects from that of group psychotherapy or group therapy groups. The primary emphasis is working with the "normal" or basically healthy individual. Such individuals may, however, be suffering some form of crisis, either situational or normal growth and development crisis. Situational crises may be those that result from illness, disease, or accidents, or from any combination of these, whereas growth and developmental crises refer to those crises that arise from inadequate or borderline adaptation to the requirements of a current psychosocial stage of development. Either type of crisis incurs certain emotional reactions that may be painful and distressing to the individual, but which, generally speaking, if the individual is supported and counseled in this crisis period, do not progress to severe emotional disorders.

Because this focus deals with "preserving" mental health versus treating full-fledged mental illness, it is appropriate that it also be described as an educative and preventative measure versus a treatment measure per se. Essentially, therapeutic groups are concerned with preventing further psychological deterioration and with educating, in the broad sense, individuals so that normal adjustment to situational and developmental crises will ensue. The assumption underlying this focus—that these groups are a form of primary prevention—is based on the fact that many mental illnesses can be prevented and "proper" functioning improved through meeting stress situations early. NOTE: Certain client groups have been identified in the literature as most in need of such primary prevention measures. Williams[16] indicates the following priority of needs: juvenile delinquency, aging, maternal and child health, school health, mental health in education, nursing, correctional and penal systems, family services, hospital and medical facilities rehabilitation, local health services, and chronic disease.

For the most part the types of therapeutic groups discussed here will be those that deal with clients in crisis on a primary prevention basis. Because these groups appear in agencies and settings that are not specifically mental health oriented, they are more likely to involve leadership by personnel with varied backgrounds. Such personnel may include, for example, general duty nurses on medical-surgical units, public health nurses, school nurses, and geriatric nurses in nursing homes and in convalescent hospitals.

The benefits to be derived from therapeutic groups for clients in crisis are numerous. Benefits for the physically ill may include adaptation to hospitalization and illness. The individual's reaction to physical illness or to such impairments of bodily functions as loss of limb or visual handicaps is typically a negative one. His ability to maintain his dignity in light of former impressions of himself and his capabilities is hampered. A group experience in which he can compare himself with others who are similarly handicapped and in which he can share his frustrations is extremely helpful in his working through his present situational crisis so that he will develop more positive feelings about himself and about his unexpected future. Patients who are anticipating surgery may experience a decrease in disabling anxiety when in a group experience they benefit from others revealing and receiving feedback about fears they themselves did not acknowledge. Groups with cancer patients and their families reduce patients' anxieties that are sometimes fostered by misconceptions and prevent the isolation patients feel when faced with alterations in body image, lifestyle, and prospects of dying.

Groups in the community in such formal agencies as clinics or in informal settings like neighborhood or youth groups can be a potential resource for problem solving and education. Groups with unwed mothers or delinquent youth, for example, can provide sound advice as well as emotional support.

Groups with youth in the schools and with the aged in nursing homes can provide still additional benefits. These groups may deal more specifically with growth and developmental crises. With the aged these groups offer an important alternative to complete social disengagement. With youth they offer a source of support and guidance that would not otherwise be available in the home, in the typical classroom, or in the peer group.

Nurse-led groups of adolescents and children have been geared to providing information as well as role modeling and creating an atmosphere of interest, objectivity, and tolerance—an atmosphere that may be in direct contrast to that which they experience in school, in peer groups, or in their homes. Information and advice can be as varied as sex and drug education materials and how to express feelings and preferences to persons in authority.

The selection of persons for therapeutic group experiences seems at first to obey no particular criteria. Anyone could, it may be said, benefit from such a group experience. Although there is some truth to this assertion, it is important to consider that such groups do offer unique contributions and that their uniqueness should not be obscured if they are to be utilized most efficiently. These groups, needless to say, would not be appropriate for patients whose primary problem is mental illness, regardless of the fact that such patients are found in many nonpsychiatric agencies. It is important to stress this point, since there is a definite temptation to include these patients in any form of mental health endeavor. In addition, patients who would otherwise be good candidates for such groups but who are temporarily inaccessible should not be included. Such persons would include, for example, the immediately postoperative patient and the acutely physically ill. The mode of interaction most appropriate in these instances would involve one-to-one relationship approaches. In the community at large, persons who are seeking optimal growth and awareness are not good candidates for these groups. It is frequently the case that these individuals have adapted adequately to their current stage of psychosocial development but wish to extend certain areas of psychosocial growth. Groups appropriate to these persons will be examined in detail in the chapter on awareness and sensitivity groups.

Groups with medical-surgical patients

Therapeutic groups may be employed with a variety of general hospital patients. The decision to confine this discussion primarily to the patient on medical-surgical units is intended to call attention to the fact that emotional phenomena should be considered important in the treatment of patients with frank physiological disorders and to explore the relatively recent use of group work by nurses in an area that has been virtually neglected by mental health professionals.

Therapeutic groups on these units as well as in other rehabilitation and treatment centers deal with a variety of patient types. Some of these types include patients who are physically disabled, infectious, preoperative, postoperative, and those for whom hospitalization is a regulative measure. Group work with the chronically physically ill—stroke patients, aphasiacs, the blind, multiple sclerosis victims, epileptics, and diabetics—is described in the literature. Group work with preoperative patients, for example, for elective abdominal surgery, was found to be quite successful with respect to uncovering concerns and instructing patients.[11] Group work with tuberculosis patients represents a more long-standing use of therapeutic groups with medical problems.

For the most part, leaders of therapeutic groups with medical-surgical patients have held two essentially different perspectives about the purpose of these groups. Some leaders focus on modifying disruptive behavior of these patients on the unit;

others focus, more indirectly, on alleviating stress due to hospitalization and illness.[9] The former approach strives to modify what is assumed to be preexisting psychological illness exacerbated by the presence of physical illness or disability. The latter approach makes no pretense about correcting for preexisting psychological illness, nor does it assume that there is a preexisting illness inherent in the patient's current adaptation. This approach characteristically strives for a change in perception and a decrease in disabling anxiety and frustration with the concomitant expectation that a member's potentials and capacities for effective coping and interaction with those around him will be forthcoming. This approach may also incorporate family members in the group of patients, primarily because family members are often involved in patients' concerns, indirectly and directly, and often affect their ability to cope.

Although these approaches do vary, they share a number of common features. Both approaches tend to emphasize the need to help patients work through present stress situations versus long-range in-depth analysis of the patient's psychological manifestations. Both approaches recognize the difficulty staff on units have in coping with emotional problems of patients and seek to alleviate disruptive behavior either directly as in the former approach or indirectly as in the latter. Both approaches also tend to stress renewed or increased capacity to effectively cope with a change in role or altered lifestyle. The difference in these approaches lies in how each would implement these objectives for patients. The former would consider modifying behavior; the latter, alleviating anxiety and frustration over one's illness and hospitalization.

In addition to these basic objectives of group work with medical-surgical patients, several more specific benefits accrue with regard to what seems to be these patients' unique needs and concerns. Disabled patients, for example, would seem to benefit from opportunities to develop more positive feelings about themselves in relation to their disability and to their altered future. Manaster[10] notes that in a group setting, which allows the disabled to explore feelings with others who have similar disabilities, these patients move more easily toward regarding themselves as human beings with dignity.

Groups with infectious patients would seem to be extremely important from a socializing viewpoint. Infectious patients, for instance, those in certain stages of tuberculosis, are isolated from their usual everyday life social experiences with friends, family, and associates. Such isolation or social deprivation may be extremely stressful to them. Group involvement with other tuberculosis patients not only can meet their needs for social interaction and relationships but also can afford them the opportunity of sharing similar concerns.

Preoperative patients are known to experience general anxiety and stress due to their anticipation of the pain, discomfort, and other perceived outcomes of surgery—some of which are not realistically based. Group work with these patients, as was found by Mezzanotte,[11] tended to bring to the surface fears that individual patients may not have acknowledged if these fears had not been brought up in the group discussion. These groups were also found to be helpful in instructing patients as to what to expect postoperatively; patients were found to recall and to use the instructions they received in these group discussions.

Groups with patients who have regulative medical problems, for example, diabetics and cardiac patients, may be extremely helpful in encouraging patients to respect the limitations imposed on them by their illness. In a group where there are other patients who have experienced adjustment problems, they are likely to gain increased insight into their own problems in accepting the limitations of their illness. It is often the case that staff are impatient and antagonistic to these patients because they have not followed their specific medical regimen. Patients under these circumstances would tend to experience greater feelings of acceptance and understanding if they could confront staff within a patient group experience where there are others who have also failed to meet the requirements of their treatment regimen.

Many problems confront nurses who wish to incorporate a group approach to medical-surgical patients into settings where such practices are not totally conducive to nor part of the treatment tradition. These problems, however, are not insurmountable; this fact is evident from the increasing use of such groups in various hospitals throughout the country. One problem seems to be the immobility of some patients and the typical physical arrangements of the ward. How is it possible to get patients together in a small group? Some leaders have bypassed this problem by confining their group to only ambulatory patients or to those that can be wheeled without too much difficulty to a central location—to a solarium or patient lounge. The possibility of holding small group meetings on the unit in such places as a four-bed room is still another approach and allows the leader to include less ambulatory patients. In some instances the latter approach necessitates special grouping of patients in a room, as all diabetic patients in a single room. Groups of this kind would provide for homogeneous grouping of patients as to needs and problems. It becomes clear, however, to those interested in leading these groups in this way that major structural rearrangements may be warranted on these units.

A second problem also relates to the difficulty of getting patients together, more specifically, of getting the same patients together at the same time. Both the turnover of patients on these wards and their various schedules for treatments and diagnostic tests make continuity of the therapeutic group experience difficult. Most leaders adjust to these realities by making their group open ended; that is, they accept new and any members regularly if these members are interested in attending the meetings. This is probably the most realistic solution, since making groups closed would result in few meetings with a small number of patients. Making these groups closed or open, however, has not been sufficiently tested for limitations and advantages. It is possible that the infrequent meetings with a small number of patients may be more meaningful and less frustrating to patients than larger groups with many new patients, a situation that requires much reorientation activity at each session. A decision of this kind would necessarily involve consideration of the nurse's schedule, the purpose of the group (the benefits to patients believed will come from such an experience), the number of patients available for the group experience, and the typical schedules of group members.

A final problem, which is not totally unrelated to the first two, is that these wards traditionally have been focused more precisely on the treatment of the patients' physical illness or disability with only minor attention to the emotional components of the patient's illness and adaptation. Staff have frequently not been prepared, nor do they have the time, to be concerned with patients' emotional welfare. Frequently they are out of tune with their own reactions to patients; this may lead to individual staff member withdrawal from patients who exhibit emotional stress, as well as to large-scale staff avoidance of considering the emotional side of patient care. Group leaders because of their association with the social-emotional side of patient care often encounter ambivalent feelings. On the one hand they may be welcomed with relief and sometimes unrealistic expectations; yet on the other hand, they may be avoided or sometimes prohibited because they represent the feared and uncharted territory of patient care. Nurses who seek to define their role as group leaders on these wards must be aware of possible reactions of staff and consider their rapport with staff to be just as important as that with their patient group. Some leaders have successfully minimized this problem because they were full-time regular staff members as well. Other leaders have confronted the problem more directly in their attempts to define a unique role. Note that even when leaders are regular staff members they still have the problem of helping staff accept their new activities; on top of this, they must manipulate an already demanding work schedule to make time for their group meetings. A successful approach if the leaders choose to define their role as unique seems to be to schedule informal meetings with staff to explain their activities and to listen to staff concerns about the consequences of their activities. Several leaders have found that, at least in the beginning, meetings with staff have occupied a great deal of their time on the ward. Nurses will do well to remember that in this situation, although their role is unique, they are not completely autonomous units but members of the total staff or treatment team. They have the responsibility of reporting periodically and even of justifying their decisions and activities to the rest of the staff. In addition, it is helpful if they also seek supervision of their activities from either a member of the staff or some experienced professional outside the staff group.

Groups with the aged

Group work with the aged in nursing homes and convalescent and general hospitals has received increasing attention in the last two decades. Unfortunately, as is true of therapeutic groups with most clients, the literature furnishes little systematic descriptive evidence of their use, their limitations, or their benefits. Still, it is quite evident that the therapeutic group approach has definitely taken hold in a number of diverse occupational groups as a method of working with the elderly. Burnside[2] noted that such groups have been conducted by nurses, recreational, occupational, and physical therapists, psychologists, social workers, psychiatrists, and directors of convalescent hospitals.

These groups have dealt with a range of patients from 45 to 85 years of age. The need to attend to the very old, generally those between 90 and 100 years old, has become a focus of more recent concern to leaders of these groups.[13] Patients in these groups have also varied in the nature of their disabilities and in the degree to which they were disabled. Some groups have been conducted exclusively with chronic brain syndrome patients. Other groups have included patients with such relatively heterogeneous medical problems as Parkinson's disease, pulmonary disease, cerebrovascular accidents, and multiple sclerosis.

The single most important goal assigned to these groups has been remotivation, for instance, to stimulate interaction between the aged and to help group members renew their sense of independence. Essentially these groups address themselves to the problems of social disengagement that often accompany growing dependency on others and the loss of significant others in the patients' lives. A predominant philosophy regarding the aging process and permeating leaders' attitudes toward these patients seems to be that social disengagement in the elderly can be normal and natural. It is not unhealthy for all, but for some it is a process that may lead to severe patterns of withdrawal, increased dependency, and severe depression. In the latter case, social disengagement should be discouraged. Relatively speaking, improved social relations among the aged are felt to be quite helpful regardless of the fact that a member's social disengagement is more normal than abnormal. Improved social relations are believed to give more meaning and satisfaction to the aged. Characteristically the aged are faced with a number of losses that may foster increased apprehension or resignation or both. The losses they may experience include loss of a spouse, close friends, memory and mental acuity, economic security, dignity, independence, familial surroundings, work, and feelings of usefulness.[1] In addition, they face changes in their body image and certain physical crises. Each of these experiences is by itself traumatic; considered together, they are heavy burdens to bear at an age in which one's will or energy to confront problems directly has slackened.

The benefits to individuals in these groups seem to be numerous and varied, from improving attitudes about oneself to facilitating communication and alleviating the effects of social isolation. Frequently the health and welfare problems of members as well as their feelings about loss of loved ones are discussed in these groups. Burnside[3] in her weekly group meetings with regressed, long-hospitalized convalescent patients devised various ways of decreasing the sensory impoverishment of members. Stangle[15] and others found that group discussion does much to stimulate members' thinking processes and widen their viewpoints. Shere[13] with a group of mentally fit aged—85 and over—noted the following benefits: (1) increased self-respect, (2) diminished feelings of loneliness and depression, (3) reactivated desires for social exchange, (4) reawakening of intellectual pursuits, and (5) development of capabilities for resuming community life. NOTE: The reader may have noticed how frequently the prefix *re* occurs in terminology describing the objectives and benefits of group work with the aged. The connotation here seems to be that much of the capacity currently lacking in the aged is not altogether absent; it is inactive, and given a particular social environment much of the former level of functioning of these individuals can be returned to them.

Providing an environment in which the aged can realize these benefits is not without problems, as many group leaders have noted. Some of these problems deal with the group leader's difficulty in leading these groups and in achieving gratification from them. Shere[13] noted that it was important for the group leader to assume an active role, to provide the group with leadership and a source of continuing stimulation, and to have patience and perseverance. Several other group leaders, including Shore[14] and Burnside,[2] noted that the health problems of members—their particular illnesses and diminishing faculties—challenge the imagination of the leader. Warmth and the willingness to listen, to be accepting and nonjudgmental, and to respect the process of aging were found to contribute to the ease with which these leaders established rapport and met their goals for members in their group.

Groups with schoolchildren and school personnel

Developmental crises are sometimes displayed as "learning" problems with school age persons. Such problems concern teachers, guidance counselors, psychologists, social workers, and school nurses at every level of education—primary, secondary, and collegiate. The use of group work in the schools, particularly in junior and senior high schools, has grown increasingly in the last decade. Still, there is much concern that the many difficulties manifested by these adolescents develop before they enter secondary school, a concern that has stimulated the use of group counseling at the elementary level as well.

The problems with which these groups deal are multiple and include drug abuse, sex education, learning defects, and racial tensions in the school. In many cases these groups attempt to provide models of acceptable behavior and reinforce this behavior in members. Model behavior in these groups may be exhibited by an adult leader or by certain peers "planted" by the leader in the group or by both. The rationale behind providing models of acceptable behavior involves the belief that children develop a behavior repertory by interacting with others: to learn or relearn appropriate behavior some contact with others who demonstrate the desired behaviors is necessary. Hansen, Niland, and Zani[7] claim that peer models are more effective than adult models, since students tend naturally to emulate peers.

In addition to altering behavior via provision of models, another technique that has been employed with many adolescent groups is that of helping members understand the behavioral choices open to them and the consequences of choosing one behavior over another. The assumption underlying this approach is that, given the opportunity to discuss alternative behaviors and their respective consequences, pupils will make more mature judgments, which in turn will result in more acceptable behavior. Both the use of models of acceptable behavior and of examination of behavior have been favorite techniques in groups of drug abusers, unwed pregnant girls, and those exhibiting behavior problems in the classroom.

Most leaders of these groups agree that some alternative to the classroom experience is needed by more and more students. The feeling is that too often in the classroom, emotional concerns of students are put aside so that the teacher may complete a lesson. Under these conditions students are constantly being curbed and controlled as well as being evaluated. Even children with high learning potential may be afflicted by some self-doubt and repressed aggression. Pichl[12] found that groups of children as young as 7 to 11 years of age could benefit from groups that suspend the rigidity of the classroom and offer students an alternative supervised group experience.

The use of groups with the "culturally deprived" students presents still further potentials for group work in the schools. Duncan and Gazda[5] with a group of culturally deprived, white, ninth-grade boys and girls found that these students benefited from the support and guidance given by interested others outside their socioeconomic group. They found these children typically demonstrate (1) a general lack of identification with the school and its goals, (2) a pattern of employing inappropriate means to gain acceptance and recognition, (3) a philosophy of life geared toward immediate gratification, and (4) negative identification with parental models. They suggest that a group counseling approach may be an effective means to deal with the dilemma students face, to effectively integrate them into a situation where others differ in social class background, and to help them to identify with more acceptable life goals.

Many professionals interested in the use of these groups in the schools have considered the relative value of including parents and school personnel in these groups. Some suggest that the inclusion of parents is both important and helpful. Pichl[12] explains that parallel meetings with parents of behavior problem children, aged 7 to 11 years, are advisable if lasting effects on the child's improvement are to be achieved. Involving the parents in this way tends to relieve the child of feelings of being victimized; it also reduces the separation between school administrators, teachers, children, and parents. Parental involvement in parallel groups was also found to minimize the parents' feelings of failure and enhance the school's appreciation of the family influence.

Group leaders are more likely to disagree about the use of other school personnel in parallel meetings or in the group itself. Most leaders want to secure an environment in which students feel there is little or no threat in revealing unacceptable behaviors or ideas; some students believe the inclusion of school personnel increases the threat that what they say may be used against them. In addition, leaders are concerned with achieving an atmosphere free of structure and anxieties associated with the classroom. Inclusion of school personnel, some maintain, increases the tendency for students to project a classroomlike atmosphere on the group. Other leaders argue that inclusion of staff can be helpful, since many of the problems which concern students are enacted with teachers and principals. The opportunity to work these problems out in relation to an actual relationship is sometimes helpful for both parties. For example, teachers may learn how their behavior feeds into student problems, and students can try out alternative behaviors with the teacher.

Groups with clients in the community at large

The use of groups in the community at large has largely been in a counseling capacity. Many professionals including the clergy, social workers, public health nurses, and psychiatrists and psychologists in social and mental health agencies have led groups of this kind. Essentially these groups attempt to reach the socially displaced or potentially displaced persons in families, neighborhoods, and small communities. More specifically, clients are frequently delinquent youth groups, unwed mothers, alcoholics, or drug addicts as well as certain culturally or ethnically displaced persons who have maintained a borderline adjustment to the society in which they live. Quite often these groups are located in youth centers, homes for delinquent youth, homes for unwed mothers, neighborhood centers, churches, and in places of work.

The benefits of these groups relate to the problems of adjustment of their members. They may offer factual information about how to utilize community services as well as support and encouragement. Such groups, as Gimpel[6] and others have noted, are known to operate to prevent juvenile delinquency, to provide a means by which members can obtain factual data about health and welfare concerns, and to offer an experience of group interaction in which members learn about behavioral choices open to them.

Since generally members of these groups are alienated from the mainstream of society, many of them do not have the knowledge or the power to alter their life circumstances. For example, members of a delinquent youth group may not know how to obtain legal counsel, or an unwed mother may not know what procedures to take to secure financial aid. In the case of the ethnically displaced person, knowledge of how to secure protection of his rights under the law may not be accessible to him. Such problems involving a lack of information and the need for counsel are frequently the topics of concern in these groups. Providing such factual information can be helpful in encouraging and supporting members who live, in what seems to them, an otherwise strange and hostile environment.

Because these groups operate to bring numbers of displaced persons together, they are potential sources of acceptance and understanding for persons in the community. Members are less fearful that others will condemn them or apply discrimination to them in their interactions within the group. Also, it is frequently the case that although members may share common concerns, they will differ in their ability to adapt. The strengths of members can be utilized as examples to help others meet the same problems. Members as well as the group leader may represent a more healthy or successful model to emulate. Cochran[4] notes that contrary to popular opinion, deviant life styles may not be the accepted way of life for these members. Even displaced persons seek status, recognition, and a favored response from the community. Often it is a question of learning the appropriate behavior—in this case through providing a model.

Groups in the community at large are likely to present some special problems to the nurse. The most important perhaps relates to the fact that in certain respects the nurse is an "outsider." This fact adversely affects the nurse's capacity to gain entry to preexisting groups and to transcend the barriers to effective communication with these persons once the nurse has gained entrance. Many displaced persons fear and condemn symbols of the adult social world from which they are alienated.

Often nurses may be perceived as such symbols. The greater their tendency to project their own values on group members, the more likely they are to fail in establishing rapport and a helping relationship with these persons. When clients are of a lower socioeconomic level or of a different racial group, the barriers to effective communication between them and the nurse may be even greater. On the other hand, because nurses are often genuinely interested in people and in helping if they can, but also because they possess knowledge about health and welfare concerns, they are likely to gain access to these groups more quickly and easily than can many other professionals.

REFERENCES

1. Burnside, I. M.: Loss: a constant theme in group work with the aged, Hosp. Community Psychiatry **21:**173-177, 1970.
2. Burnside, I. M.: Group work with the aged: selected literature, Gerontologist **10:**241-246, 1970.
3. Burnside, I. M.: Sensory stimulation: an adjunct to group work with the disabled aged, Ment. Hyg. **53:**381-388, 1969.
4. Cochran, M. L., and Yeaworth, R. C.: Ward meetings for teen-age mothers, Am. J. Nurs. **67:**1044-1047, 1967.
5. Duncan, J. A., and Gazda, G. M.: Significant content of group counseling sessions with culturally deprived ninth grade students, Personnel Guidance J. **46:**11-16, 1967.
6. Gimpel, H. S.: Group work with adolescent girls, Nurs. Outlook **16:**46-48, 1968.
7. Hansen, J. C., Niland, T. M., and Zani, L. P.: Model reinforcement in group counseling with elementary school children, Personnel Guidance J. **47:**741-744, 1969.
8. Holzman, S., and Sobel, N.: Improving the morale of the patients and the staff in a geriatric institution by a supervised visiting program, Gerontologist **8:**29-33, 1968.
9. Langlois, P.: Discussion, San Francisco, October 1970, University of California Medical Center.
10. Manaster, A.: The therognostic group in a rehabilitation center for the visually handicapped. In Golden Gate Group Psychotherapy Society: Summary of papers, San Francisco, 1969, The Society.
11. Mezzanotte, E. J.: Group instruction in preparation for surgery, Am. J. Nurs. **70:**89-91, 1970.
12. Pichl, W.: Group therapy with latency age children in school settings. In Golden Gate Group Psychotherapy Society: Summary of papers, San Francisco, 1969, The Society.
13. Shere, E.: Group work with the very old. In Kastenbaum, R., editor: New thoughts on old age, New York, 1964, Springer Publishing Co.
14. Shore, H.: Content of the group experience in a home for the aged, social group work with older people, New York, 1963, National Association of Social Workers.
15. Stangle, E.: Geriatric psychiatry and social psychiatry, J. Am. Geriatr. Soc. **17:**612-617, 1969.
16. Williams, R.: Trends in community psychiatry indirect services and the problem of balance in mental health programs. In Bellak, L., editor: Handbook of community mental health, New York, 1964, Grune & Stratton, p. 350.

SUGGESTED READINGS
Introduction

Berkovitz, I., editor: Adolescents grow in groups, New York, 1975, Brunner/Mazel.
Fidler, J. W.: The relationship of group psychotherapy to "therapeutic" group approaches, Int. J. Group Psychother. **20:**473-494, 1970.

Groups with medical-surgical patients

Abramson, M.: Group treatment of families of burn-injured patients, Soc. Casework **56:**235-241, 1975.

Adsett, C. A., and Bruhn, J. G.: Short-term group psychotherapy for post-myocardial infarction patients and their wives, Can. Med. Assoc. J. **99:**577-584, 1968.

Blyth, Z.: Group treatment for handicapped children, J. Psychiatr. Nurs. **7:**172-173, 1969.

Davidson, P., and Noyes, R.: Psychiatric nursing consultation on a burn unit, Am. J. Nurs. **73:**1715-1718, 1973.

Heller, U.: Handicapped patients talk together, Am. J. Nurs. **70:**332-335, 1970.

Kakkola, L., et. al.: The experimental use of discussion groups among the patients of a general hospital, Sairaanh **8:**78-85, 1971.

Langlois, P., and Teramoto, V.: Helping patients cope with hospitalization, Nurs. Outlook, **19:**334-336, 1971.

Linn, L.: Some aspects of a psychiatric program in a voluntary general hospital. In Bellak, L., editor: Handbook of community psychiatry and community mental health, New York, 1964, Grune and Stratton.

Menzies, I. E. P.: A case study in the functioning of social systems as a defense against anxiety: a report on a study of the nursing service of a general hospital Hum. Rel. **13:**95-121, 1960.

Mone, L. C.: Short-term group psychotherapy with post-cardiac patients, Int. J. Group Psychother. **20:**99-108, 1970.

Orodei, D., and Waite, N.: Group psychotherapy with stroke patients during the immediate recovery phase, Nurs. Digest, May-June 1975, pp. 26-29.

Piskor, B., and Paleos, I.: The group way to banish after-stroke blues, Am. J. Nurs. **68:**1500-1503, 1968.

Singler, J.: Group work with hospitalized stroke patients, Soc. Casework **56:**348354, 1975.

Smith, E. D.: Group conference for postpartum patients, Am. J. Nurs. **71:**112-113.

Groups with the aged

Cumming, E., and Genry, W. E.: Growing old—the process of disengagement, New York, 1961, Basic Books, Inc., Publishers.

Burnside, I.: Loss: a constant theme in group work with the aged, Hosp. Community Psychiatry **21:**21-25, 1970.

Klein, W. H., Le Shan, E. J., and Furman, S. S.: Promoting mental health of older people through group methods, New York, 1965, Mental Health Materials Center.

Kubie, S., and Landau, G.: Group work with the aged, New York, 1963, International Universities Press.

Levine, R. L.: Disengagement in the elderly—its causes and effects, Nurs. Outlook **17:**28-30, 1969.

Lowy, L.: Roadblocks in group work practice with older people, Gerontologist **2:**109113, 1967.

Rosin, A.: Group discussions: a therapeutic tool in a chronic diseases hospital, Geriatrics **30:**45-48, 1975.

Ross, M.: Community geriatric group therapies: a comprehensive review. In Rosenbaum, M., and Berger, M., editors: Group psychotherapy and group function, ed. 2, New York, 1975, Basic Books, Inc., Publishers.

Rustin, S. L., and Wolk, R. L.: The use of specialized group psychotherapy techniques in a home for the aged. In Moreno, J., editor: Group psychotherapy, New York, 1963, Beacon House.

Silverstein, S.: A new venture in group work with the aged, Soc. Casework **50:**573-580, 1969.

Groups with schoolchildren and school personnel

Amundson, N.: TA with elementary school children, Trans. Anal. J. **5:**247-250, 1975.

Atkeson, P., and Suttentag, M.: A parent discussion group in a nursery school, Soc. Casework **56:**515-520, 1975.

Barnes, G.: Deprived adolescents, a use of group work, Br. J. Soc. Work **5:**149-160, 1975.

Berkovitz, I., editor: When schools care: creative use of groups in secondary schools, New York, 1975, Brunner/Mazel.

Brocker, T.: Group methods in parent education, Int. J. Group Psychother. **25:**315-321, 1975.

Bulton, L.: Development group work with adolescents, New York, 1975, Holsted Press.

Corbett, J., and Roberts, P. R.: Reclaiming the infuriated in a ghetto-area school, Am. J. Nurs. **70:**1476-1485, 1967.

Epstein, N., and Altman, S.: Experiences in converting an activity group into verbal group therapy with latency-age boys, Int. J. Group Psychother. **22:**93-100, 1972.

English, R. W., and Higgins, T. E.: Client-centered group counseling with pre-adolescents, J. Sch. Health **41:**507-510, 1971.

Gitterman, A.: The school: group work in the public schools. In Schartz, W., and Zalba, S., editors: The practice of group work, New York, 1972, Columbia University Press.

Gurman, A. S.: Group counseling with underachievers, Int. J. Group Psychother. **19:**463-472, 1969.

Kelley, J. B., Samules, M., and McClurkin, L. J.: Reaching out to parents of handicapped children—a group approach in an inner city school, J. Sch. Health **44:**577-579, 1975.

Mitchell, K.: A group program for the treatment of failing college students, Behav. Ther. **6:**324-336, 1975.

Sands, R., and Golieb, S.: Breaking the bonds of tradition: a reenactment of group treatment of latency-age children, Am. J. Psychiatry **131:**662-665, 1974.

Sugar, M., editor: The adolescent in group and family therapy, New York, 1975, Brunner/Mazel.

Schmock, R., and Schmock, P.: Group processes in the classroom, ed. 2, Dubuque, Iowa, 1975, William C. Brown Co., Publishers.

Groups with clients in the community at large

Alder, J.: Therapeutic work with displaced persons, Int. J. Group Psychother. **3:**302-306, 1953.

Daniels, A. M.: Reaching unwed adolescent mothers, Am. J. Nurs. **69:**332-336, 1969.

Farris, B., Murillo, G., and Hall, W.: The neighborhood. In Schwartz, W., and Zalba, S., editors: The practice of group work, New York, 1972, Columbia University Press.

Reiser, M.: A drop-in group for teenagers in a poverty area. In Berkovitz, I., editor: Adolescents grow in groups, New York, 1975, Brunner/Mazel.

Rochman, A.: Talking it out rather than fighting it out: prevention of a delinquent gang war by group therapy intervention, Int. J. Group Psychother. **19:**518-521, 1969.

Savino, A., and Sanders, R.: Working with abusive parents—group therapy and home visits, Am. J. Nurs. **73:**482-484, 1973.

Shapiro, J.: Single-room occupancy group work with urban rejects in a slum hotel. In Schwartz, W., and Zalba, S., editors: The practice of group work, New York, 1972, Columbia University Press.

CHAPTER 3

Self-help groups

Introduction

Self-help groups, as opposed to therapeutic groups and group psychotherapy groups, are for the most part organized and operated by group members themselves without the supervision, guidance, or leadership of professionally trained group leaders. Characteristically they intend to solve the problems of members as defined by members. An attitude of "we 'know' best" what the problems of members are and what will work in relieving stress, as well as a certain mistrust and lack of confidence in alternative, more traditional regimens, permeates much of the philosophy of such organized self-help groups as Alcoholics Anonymous (AA), Synanon, women's groups, Parents Anonymous, and self-help health groups. Essentially, self-help groups may be said to be groups of, for, and by the client. When and if professionals do participate in group meetings, they do so by invitation and are placed in an ancillary role.

As conceived of here, self-help groups include many types of formal and informal groupings (or subcultures). They are usually organized for some specific purpose, which reflects members' problems with, for example, a lifestyle that is undesirable or which reflects members' needs for adjustment to an alien environment. Individuals who have addictions to drugs, food, or alcohol have in some ways utilized these groups to aid them in altering their lifestyles. Persons who have suffered some loss of bodily function or who have acquired some handicap, for example, because of necessary surgery, have formulated clubs that enable them to adapt more successfully to their disabilities. Also, persons faced with commitment to new and alien environments, for instance, through institutionalization in a school or in a hospital, or faced with return to an alien environment, for example, after discharge from a mental hospital or a prison, seek refuge in self-help groups.

Self-help groups are not new in the array of possible therapeutic activities open to individuals with special problems. The tendency for persons with similar concerns and needs to group themselves together to combat their common problem is as old as mankind itself. The success and pervasiveness of such groups, however, might well vary from society to society, depending on the attitudes of professionals toward groups that operate outside their control and supervision and in competition with their professional services. In the United States alone, such groups as Alcoholics Anonymous and Synanon have gained increased recognition and acceptance by the health care industry, yet they are still questioned by many health professionals as well as by local citizens who do not approve of the somewhat unorthodox approaches utilized by these groups.

In spite of this opposition, throughout the last quarter of a century such self-help groups as Alcoholics Anonymous, Synanon, and TOPS (Take Off Pounds Sensibly) have become a popular and pervasive feature of the treatment and rehabilitation of alcoholics, drug addicts, and overweight persons. Likewise, organizations for persons who have undergone such operations as colostomy or laryngectomy have sprung up within many communities. Part of the popularity of currently existing self-help groups comes from the fact that they have been quite successful in effecting "cures" or meeting members' needs, over and above the success of therapeutic approaches used prior to this time. To some extent even health professionals are willing to concede that these groups have much to offer and recommend that their own clients join these groups as an adjunct to professional care. Still some professionals are concerned that they will be accused of abrogating their responsibility by turning the job of treatment over to such groups.[4]

The focus of self-help groups is for the most part different from that of group psychotherapy and therapeutic groups. Their chief aims are to (1) control member behavior, (2) ameliorate stress due to common problems, for example, by giving advice and sharing coping strategies, and (3) maintain member self-esteem and legitimacy in the face of societal pressure. They are not equipped nor do they intend to focus on furthering members' insight, on personality reconstruction, or on education per se. Chiefly their focus is on repression of impulses and promoting of socialization. Alcoholics Anonymous, Synanon, and TOPS attempt to curb and repress directly the impulses of members to succumb to their addictions. Their success in helping members repress their impulses largely results from the group norms and sanctions applied to differentiate "good" and "bad" members. To be a "good" member, and essentially in order to belong, one must not drink, take drugs, or overeat, respectively.

In addition to a focus on repression of impulses these groups focus on socialization of members. The socialization that goes on in these groups is a process not only of meeting members' needs for social contact with others but also of instilling certain perspectives and values in members. To be successful in aiding members to adapt to new environments or to give up destructive habits, self-help groups must use specific ways in socializing members so that they accept the norms and perspectives of the group. Group ceremonies such as initiation processes often are good examples of the socialization methods that these groups will use. In turn the group promises to fulfill members' needs to socialize with others who are facing similar problems. Professionals who have visited various types of self help groups are cognizant of the importance of the socialization processes that go on in the group. Many social science theorists who have observed the socialization that goes on within inmate cultures in institutions claim that this process is essential and is aimed at opposing the formal institutional rules and regulations, the outcome being that members of the subculture are able to maintain former identities in this new and alien environment.

Self-help groups, as has been suggested, can be of either a formal (organized) or informal (ad hoc) variety. They may operate out of health institutions, as do many colostomy and laryngectomy clubs and some Alcoholics Anonymous groups, or they may operate at large in the community, for example, in makeshift club houses as does Synanon. Also they may operate within existing institutions as do, for instance, inmate subcultures in schools, hospitals, and prisons. Some of these groups that operate in the larger community actually provide residential facilities for their members. Most groups will in any case provide for frequent contacts with other members. In large metropolitan areas an alcoholic or drug addict may attend a group meeting any day or night of the week. Telephone calls or visits from members to other members at any time are also provided. Part of the success and desirability of these groups is no doubt related to the fact that contact with other members at any time is possible and encouraged.

Although the benefits of these groups are quite varied, the following seem to be quite important to members: support and empathic understanding, impetus to change, and knowledge of how to "work the system." Empathy and understanding by other members is quite supportive to the members of Alcoholics Anonymous, for example. With the addict, the alcoholic, and the overweight person in particular, feelings of isolation and loneliness are acute. Actual prejudice and disapproval from others outside the group cause the member to have serious doubts about ever really "fitting" into the society at large. Still they realize that former acquaintances are not helpful if they wish to change their lifestyles. Because these groups contain persons who themselves face or have faced similar problems and who also are attempting to change or adapt, they are a source of comfort and support. In the group, members are assured of the necessary empathy and understanding that assists them in the process of changing and adapting.

Closely linked with the benefit of support and empathic understanding that members receive in these groups is the impetus to change that is fostered in the group. Role models play an important part with regard to this benefit. Role models in self-help groups essentially reinforce the desired lifestyle or means of adaptation valued by the group. Role models in Alcoholics Anonymous, for example, are those persons who have sufficiently maintained sobriety as a way of living. Role models in inmate subcultures are those who have demonstrated an ability to not be totally incorporated by the goals of the formal institution and who have acquired a certain amount of skill and knowledge to "work the system." The success of others that is demonstrated by role models who have themselves faced the same problems tends to increase members' confidence that they can adapt or change too.

A benefit that is probably more associated with subculture self-help groups in institutions is that related to "working the system." "Working the system" merely means that individuals manipulate the formal rules and regulations of the institution to meet their needs as unique individuals within settings that treat all inmates the same. In any institution the ability to "work the system" includes very different capacities. As a member of the inmate culture one learns the specific skills and knowledges necessary to work that particular system.

The nature of members' concerns and needs in self-help groups becomes quite clear from this discussion. Members are faced with the problems of changing their lifestyles either to incorporate new behaviors and disregard old habits or to incorporate a way of life appropriate to the new and foreign environment to which they have been admitted—quite often involuntarily. They anticipate failure to adjust to a new lifestyle or fear that their adjustment will result in a loss of sense of self. Persons who have not or are not experiencing these same concerns cannot provide adequate support and comfort. Alone, these persons feel powerless; together with those who share their concerns, their hope for adjustment is restored. Proof that change is possible and that others have succeeded is crucial, especially when their own self-discipline is involved in the adjustment process. The success of the group itself in aiding an individual's adjustment is important to members. Partaking in the group to help others—the demonstrated success of the group—enhances the individual member's self-esteem and provides him with added confidence to face his own problems of adjustment.

In light of the nature of members' problems and needs and in light of the benefits that self-help groups seem to provide members, the role of the nurse as a trained professional in such groups is not entirely clearcut or straightforward. It has already been noted that the empathy and increased sense of confidence that can be derived from self-help group experiences are largely a result of the fact that the group is made up only of those who share the common problem, that is, that the group excludes professional leaders. It is questionable whether a professional could or should ever be considered an actual "member." Likewise there is sufficient data to indicate that the best leadership for the group is that which mobilizes the members' own capacities to lead on the basis of their personal success with reference to the goals of the group. What then is the role of the nurse, a knowledgeable professional, yet, clearly, a "nonmember"?

The role of the nurse would seem to encompass at least two major functions: (1) that of verifying the success of individuals and the group as a whole, (2) that of identifying and referring persons to these groups, and (3) that of providing knowledge—such as would a resource person—about the social systems with which members must deal and the variety of problems and needs that are primary or secondary to the group's major concern. The first function relates to the fact that recognition and approval from the "establishment" can fortify members' and the group's confidence. It is not entirely true that these groups and the individuals within these groups can go without the approval and support of more orthodox treatment and rehabilitation personnel and organizations. Such approval and support to some extent lend added confidence and recognition to these groups and quite frequently lead to new members' joining these groups. There is no question that the nurse can provide important services to these groups by referring clients or by bolstering the group's own self-image through the nurse's approval.

Nurses' experience and knowledge of health problems, as well as their knowledge of how institutions function, are unique to the group. The various concerns of members often reflect inadequate information in both areas, partly due to their lack of professional training and partly due to the fact that members do not occupy positions of authority in the institutions that affect them.

The role of nurses as resource persons and as persons who can verify and support the success of the self-help group, then, seems to be fairly clearcut. Their role as traditional therapists or group leaders, however, would seem to be limited as well as inadvisable.

Informal subgroups in institutions

Self-help groups, as they are conceived here, include informal subgroups of clients or inmates in a variety of total or quasi institutions, for example, the school, the hospital, and the prison.[1] Members in each of these instances are expected to adapt to a new or alien environment in which change in their behavior, attitudes, self-image, and even physical appearance are forthcoming and may be expected. Quite frequently, members' admissions to these institutions have been mandatory and involuntary, although the outcomes of the institutional experience may not be totally undesirable to the individual.

The inmate or subculture groups in these institutions have been described extensively by many sociologists and social psychologists. Among the most renown is the portrayal by Erving Goffman in his book, *Asylums*.[2] Total institutions, as Goffman describes them, are in the business of transforming clients; groups of people are processed together, categorized, and subjected to some uniform application of a procedure that does something for the clients. To accomplish this aim the institution utilizes certain techniques, as stripping incoming clients of all former objects of identity. Inmates necessarily experience a sense of self-mortification and role dispossession along with feelings that they are no longer "their own men." The inmate or client subculture allows its members to retain a sense of uniqueness and at the same time provides them with the support they need in adjusting to this alien environment.

Fellow inmates know and understand the devastating experiences of institutionalization, for they have undergone or are currently undergoing the same experiences. Many of them have successfully adjusted while still maintaining a sense of uniqueness. These members are quite often the role models and leaders of the group who give others the confidence that they too might achieve some form of acceptable adjustment—both in terms of the institution's goals and in terms of their own needs not to succumb entirely to the institutional regime. In hospitals these leaders may be those members who take it on themselves to visit the newcomers in order to orient them to the hospital routine, the authority system, and the possible outcome of his experience in surgery or in therapy with certain psychiatrists. In schools these leaders may have inside information about the courses and instructors or even, who to see to get drugs. In prisons they are members who may have obtained special bargaining power with the guards and who negotiate with the new inmates to provide them with "protection" or special favors.

It is obvious that although the services rendered by these groups and their leaders are not altogether desirable to either the individual or to the institution, the support and understanding that these groups and their leaders provide are crucial to members' adjustments to the institution and in light of their needs to maintain a separate identity in an impersonal, processing system.

In addition to the support and understanding that these groups provide, the knowledge of how to "work the system" is perhaps an equally valuable benefit to members. Quite often the members of these subgroups have a keen sense of the nature of the formal and informal communication and authority structures that exist within the institution. Also, they have learned how they can deviate from existing rules to achieve some sense of autonomy and self-mastery. "Working the system" may in some instances include such things as obtaining forbidden satisfactions or making secondary adjustments so that one does not succumb totally to the goals of the institution. Its merit lies in the fact that members do achieve a sense of self-control and individual identity despite the institution's attempts to process them irrespective of their unique identity.

The business of incorporating various members of "the establishment," including such trained professionals as nurses, in these groups is extremely difficult and not altogether sound. In most cases members of these groups do not want, or allow, members of the establishment to interfere with the group's activities. In some instances they attempt to keep the nature of their meetings (the content of their discussions) secret. This may be because what they do say is not totally true, is one sided, or would threaten professionals; but also, the exclusion of professionals and persons of authority in the institution allows them to develop a sense of belongingness and cohesion in the group that might not be possible if persons not in their position—who were not experiencing the same problems and concerns—were included in the group. The latter is the case with Alcoholics Anonymous and other associations that hold closed as well as open meetings. The participation of persons who do not share the same problems limits the cohesion of the group. Thus professionals' attempts to be incorporated are often blocked by members. Professionals disguised as inmates is a solution that in itself is not altogether sound. In addition, it is not clear that the incorporation of a professional or person in authority, especially if his position supersedes members' ability to relate in the group, is entirely justified if one keeps in mind the benefits these groups provide. The support, understanding, and ability to "work the system" are a result of only persons who are themselves inmates being included in the group. These benefits, although not altogether desirable in the minds of professionals or persons in authority in the institution, do seem to serve an important role in the overall adjustment of individuals to the process of institutionalization. The most obvious conclusion is that if professionals were to be included, the benefits heretofore provided to members would no longer be forthcoming. The support, understanding, and knowledge conveyed to members about how to "work the system" would be modified by the presence of these "outsiders."

The question arises: how can the nurse, a professional and sometimes a member of the establishment, establish a role that is both helpful yet unobtrusive in these groups? From this discussion it would seem that one role appropriate for nurses may be that of benevolent resource person. Otherwise they may not choose to operate as members or leaders of the group per se, but they might be called on by the group for information and support at various times. In fact, this is quite often the role that a staff nurse on a ward in a general hospital or a school nurse, for example, will assume. Nurses can establish a rapport with these groups that will create trust and will gain entrance for them at times when members feel they are needed. Nurses in general have no trouble initiating such a relationship, since they are often regarded as benevolent resource persons in networks of authority systems, such as hospitals, schools, prisons, or the community at large.

Alcoholics Anonymous and its auxiliary groups

Alcoholics Anonymous groups have sprung up in virtually every area of the country and are now prevalent not only in large cities but also in small towns and communities as well. In addition the traditional form of the group—that it usually contained an undifferentiated population of alcoholics alone—has changed. Now groups specialize in the rehabilitation of different clients in certain age groups or vary to include not only the alcoholic but his family as well. In some communities, groups have also differentiated themselves in terms of socioeconomic status. One may belong to the "uptown" or "downtown" group, or simply the "mission" group. Quite frequently groups will take on names that indicate for them a certain motive or identity above and beyond that of Alcoholics Anonymous organizations per se.

The success of Alcoholics Anonymous in keeping members "dry" is now well known and respected by many health professionals. The success of these groups over other orthodox therapies lies largely in the attributes of the groups themselves, but also in the fault of many professionals. Physicians, nurses, and other health professionals have in some cases failed at being patient, tolerant, and understanding of alcoholics. Their reluctance to attempt therapy with them has in turn resulted in a lack of trust and confidence by the alcoholic in the professional's ability to help him. Self-help groups, on the other hand, have gained the confidence and trust of the alcoholic. Made up of alcoholics themselves, these groups provide the patience, understanding, and support the alcoholic needs if he is to relinquish his habit. In addition they insist that the alcoholic resist his need to drink if he is to continue to be a member.

Members of Alcoholics Anonymous have a particular conception of alcoholism. Essentially they regard it as an incurable disease, but one which may be successfully contained if the alcoholic does not take even one drink. Other analyses of alcoholism conceptualize in depth the pattern of adaptation peculiar to alcoholics. Under the influence of stress the following process seems to be operant with the alcoholic: (1) he experiences feelings of inadequacy along with a painful awareness of reality; (2) this produces stress; (3) he compensates by drinking alcohol and experiences reduced tension; (4) this produces a quasieuphoria that does not last; (5) guilt feelings set in; and (6) the alcoholic drinks more and more to cope with his unresolved problems.[3] The compulsive drinking typical of the alcoholic causes secondary social difficulties that produce problems for himself and his family. Social, financial, and occupational, as well as physical, problems usually stem from the alcoholic's addiction. His family is beset by problems of financial support or find it difficult to be tolerant and understanding of his problems. They feel ashamed, angry, and resentful toward the alcoholic. There is usually some attempt on their part to be accepting, but this usually leads to frustration and eventually to their rejection of the alcoholic altogether. The rejection of family members merely documents for the alcoholic that which he already suspected, that is, that he is a worthless and an inadequate human being.

The role of Alcoholics Anonymous and other groups working in behalf of the alcoholic has been quite impressive in meeting the needs of the alcoholic and his family. Groups that include family members are able to offer them an opportunity to share common frustrations and to release angry feelings that they have harbored. Families are able to learn that their feelings and modes of relating to the alcoholic in the family are not totally unique. Families attempt to examine how they are involved in the alcoholic's disease and what alternatives are open to them in relating to him. Essentially, family members are helped to understand themselves and the alcoholic better.

The benefits of Alcoholics Anonymous, in particular, for the alcoholic himself can be found in a careful examination of the processes and activities of these groups. A study I[3] made in 1964 revealed that several benefits seemed to come from interaction of members in these groups. Warmth, support, empathic understanding, and unconditional acceptance seemed to permeate members' relationships with each other. These elements seemed to work to bolster the individual's sense of adequacy and self-confidence. In addition the norms of the group operated directly to repress members' compulsions to drink. The group's doctrines, for example, specify that one is always an alcoholic and that one drink is the alcoholic's downfall. Members are encouraged to accept this perspective and avoid alcohol altogether. Members are not barred from the group if they resume drinking, but if they do resume drinking, they usually are unable to face the group. If one member resumes drinking, it is a tragedy for the group as well.

Alcoholics Anonymous uses role models to further control its members' compulsions to drink and to instill confidence that sobriety is possible as well as desirable. The role models in Alcoholics Anonymous groups are usually those who have maintained sobriety over a period of time and have started "on the road back" to a more socially acceptable and financially secure level of functioning. They are able to hold down a job and sustain some form of close relationships with others. Meetings frequently feature the story of how a member came to an all-time low, sought help from Alcoholics Anonymous, and has since achieved sobriety and adapted more successfully to everyday life situations. Members applaud his success and are reminded that Alcoholics Anonymous has the right idea about alcoholism and about the steps necessary to achieve a more adequate adjustment. Because it is believed that even a successful member still possesses the disease, members can more easily identify with him and hope for their own success in the future.

The role of nurses as suggested by observations of these groups largely relies on their capacity to serve as unobtrusive resource persons. Although nurses with specialized knowledge of the psychodynamics of the alcoholic's personality and of his health and welfare problems have valuable information, they may only be able to use their skill and knowledge indirectly when members seek their advice. Yet members quite often do not have access to certain facts about their health and welfare problems and can benefit greatly from the special preparation or training nurses bring to the group.

For several reasons it would seem that their role must also be an unobtrusive one, however. As indicated previously, the success of Alcoholics Anonymous relies on the fact that all members are alcoholics who "know" and experience common concerns. The successful operation of the group depends on the quality of members' participation and involvement and not on the skill and knowledge of a professional "outsider" in leading the group. It is likely that an active role might disrupt the group's ability to instill confidence in members and to provide them with the quality of support and understanding needed.

Nonetheless, members are quite interested in the opinions and evaluations of professionals. A nurse who recognizes the potential of these groups and is convinced of their ability to help the alcoholic and his family may provide these groups with the outside support and recognition they need. In addition, members frequently harbor certain misconceptions about professionals and their attitudes toward alcoholics. Such misconceptions are the result, as well as the cause, of a relative lack of communication between Alcoholics Anonymous and more orthodox treatment professionals. The nurse can serve as an important liaison between the health professions and self-help groups for alcoholics.

Synanon groups and other organizations for the drug addict

Synanon foundations, which have developed primarily since the late 1950s, now have locations throughout the country and have become pervasive in the restoration and rehabilitation of addicts to a more normal existence. They involve everything from residential facilities to periodic group meetings and Synanon games.

The problem of keeping the addict from resuming his drug habit after an initial treatment phase, not unlike that of keeping the alcoholic from resuming his drinking, is a difficult one. Many of the orthodox treatment and rehabilitation centers, such as the public health service hospitals and county and city programs, although they provide a beginning service to addicts, are not adequate in the later phases of recovery. It has been noted that only about one-fourth of the patients admitted to hospitals of this kind are "cured" and that up to 90% of those discharged become addicted again within six months after discharge.[2] Thus the tendency for addicts to return to drug habits even after extensive treatment by health professionals is great. In part this is the result not only of a lack of sufficient follow-up care but also of the nature of the addict's commitment in the first place. Quite often the addict seeks "a cure" only because he is too ill, too old, or too poor to support his struggle to get drugs in the amounts he needs. Necessarily his commitment to a program is contingent on circumstances that in some instances are altered by a quick cure, for example, his ability to obtain money to support a habit. Quick cures can enable the addict to get a temporary job, which then provides him with enough money to start on drugs again.

Synanon groups recognize the halfhearted attempts of addicts for what they are. In many instances they will confront the addict with his insincerity and demand of him a greater commitment to a life without drugs. Essentially Synanon has been known not to accept as members those who are currently taking drugs.

The problem of drug addiction, like that of alcoholism, involves a complex pattern of compulsive behavior. Initially it has a basis in feelings of boredom, loneliness, and a desire to belong or to find relief from depression. Continued and sustained use of drugs involves more than just these feelings, however. A pattern like the following is more descriptive of the problems of the addict: (1) feelings of boredom, loneliness, and so on produce anxiety; (2) this anxiety stimulates an immature desire for escape from reality and from the responsibility of self-stimulation through drugs; (3) taking drugs gives the addict immediate relief from stress; and (4) to get the same relief repeatedly, the dose must be increased.[2] Once addicted the addict experiences an overpowering desire or need (compulsion) to continue taking the drug and to obtain it by any means. It is not unusual that he will be willing to commit crimes to obtain drugs or money to buy drugs to support his increasingly expensive habit. Secondary to his addiction are certain physical problems—malnutrition, skin infections, and toxic reactions—as well as financial crises and social-vocational incapacities that result from his drug habit.

The benefits that Synanon and other organizations of addicts seem to provide for members are quite comprehensive. Synanon is known to provide residential facilities and jobs, as well as the more intangible benefits to be gained through its group meetings and games. Synanon games in particular seem to facilitate the breaking down of the destructive defenses that cause addicts to escape through the use of drugs. The support that comes from Synanon groups does not arise from the warmth and unconditional acceptance so characteristic of Alcoholics Anonymous groups, but from the security that one cannot fool another addict and through the dependency that is allowed members in the early phases of their rehabilitation.

As in Alcoholics Anonymous, role models, who are sometimes the recognized leaders of Synanon games, are employed to a great extent to instill confidence in members so that they can stay off drugs. Overconfidence is, however, guarded against, since it either demonstrates insincerity on the part of the addict or is an example of a tendency toward unrealistic perceptions.

Synanon games, like Alcoholics Anonymous meetings, essentially are substitutions for addicts and alcoholics, respectively. In Alcoholics Anonymous meetings it was noted that members transmit feelings of warmth, acceptance, and support to one another, which produce an anesthetizing effect similar to that produced with alcohol. In Synanon games, however, the atmosphere is more intensive and stimulating, provoking feelings and confrontation between members. The exhilaration that comes from participating in these groups most certainly operates as drugs operate, in overcoming addicts' feelings of boredom and loneliness. These games are not likely, however, to give the addict the sense of euphoria and escape from reality that drugs do.

A typical Synanon game may involve the following types of interaction. Everyone in the group settles down, as comfortably as possible, in a circle facing one another. There is usually a brief silence while members seem to appraise one another. Then abruptly they launch into an intensive emotional discussion of personal problems. A keypoint in the sessions is an emphasis on extreme, uncompromising candor about one another. Everything, excluding bodily harm to one another, is permissible. The idea is to prevent members from covering up; delusions and distortions about oneself are attacked again and again by the group.

The role of nurses in Synanon, like that in Alcoholics Anonymous, may be one more of an unobtrusive resource person. Nurses must keep in mind that "playing a role" with addicts is not advisable. Their participation, whatever it may consist of, would necessitate an authentic presentation of self. Secondary to this would be their ability to assume a role as knowledgeable resource person to the group. Not every nurse would feel comfortable under these conditions. Certainly those who have successfully combined their occupational role with their own perceptions of self may feel less threatened than those who have not.

Like that of Alcoholics Anonymous, Synanon's success lies in the fact that addicts are able to help themselves in these groups. Proof that they are able to alter their drug habits on their own through the group is necessary in generating a sense of self-confidence in members. In addition, few persons other than addicts themselves would not be fooled by the games addicts play with regard to relinquishing their habits. Because nurses might not be as effective in detecting addict games and because the success of Synanon is largely due to the ability of addicts to help themselves, the role of nurses may be less dominant in these groups. Nurses do, however, possess valuable knowledge, for example, about the health problems of the addict, that would be helpful to the group. In addition they can serve as important liaisons between health facilities and these groups, for instance, in providing follow-up supervision of addicts or simply in bettering the relationships between these two services. As with Alcoholics Anonymous, health professionals tend to know very little about the operations and provisions of Synanon, and addicts tend to distort the attitudes of professionals. The nurse can do much to improve the communication between the two.

TOPS, Weight Watchers, and other weight-reducing groups

Self-help groups that are quite popular among the lay public are such weight-reducing groups or retreats as those sponsored by TOPS (Take Off Pounds Sensibly), Weight Watchers, and others. These groups can be found to operate as private organizations out of commercial establishments such as department stores or health salons. Weight-reducing groups often advertise to acquire clients.

The psychosocial problems of the overweight person are not totally different from those of the alcoholic or drug addict. Members frequently regard their eating as a habit and food as the source of their addiction. Patterns of compulsive eating resemble those of compulsive drinking and drug taking. Food addicts are known to consume food from feelings of boredom, loneliness, and inadequacy. The consumption of food gives immediate satisfaction but only temporarily relieves the anxiety of the overweight person. A compulsive need (drive) causes the food addict to consume more and more food. The addict's problems remain, and the major source of relief associated with these problems is the eating of food. As with other addicts, the food addict is psychologically dependent on his intake of food.

Weight-reducing groups provide many benefits to their members. Socialization is an important provision. Members, as it was noted, often eat out of boredom and loneliness. Weight-reducing groups often hold daily meetings. Although some of these meetings are designed to be merely weigh-in sessions, others provide extensive discussion time and lectures. Members not only benefit from the fact that these are socializing experiences, but also from the fact that the experience itself is directed toward abolishing their compulsive eating patterns. Like Alcoholics Anonymous and Synanon, role models in these groups are important. Persons who have lost a great deal of weight are often presented as keynote speakers in these groups. They describe their own problems and explain how the group has helped them. Others in the group identify with them and are instilled with new confidence in their own ability to resist overeating. (See Wagonfeld.[5])

An important facet of this interplay between role models and members is the sense of competition generated. The group seems to foster competition among members to lose weight. Members compete with others but also against their own tendencies to overeat. Competition in this case seems to give members added incentive to lose weight and repress their urge to overeat.

Despite this atmosphere of social competition, these groups seem to provide tremendous support to members. Members explain how important it is to them to be able to meet and talk with others who are trying to lose weight or who are extremely overweight. This type of support in part is generated by the feelings outside the group that one is different and distasteful to others. An emphasis on thinness in our society contributes to members' feelings of isolation from others outside the group.

The role of nurses in weight-reducing groups, like that in other self-help groups discussed thus far, is more appropriately that of unobtrusive resource persons. A sense of belonging in these groups is enhanced by the fact that all members are food addicts and overweight. In addition the success of the group depends on members' ability to help themselves. Dependence on outside professional advice, encouragement, or disapproval to relinquish one's overeating may not have worked for these individuals. Still nurses do have important knowledge and skill, for example, with regard to health problems, that are helpful to the group. Frequently these groups have adapted fixed diets or menus; the nurse can be helpful in advising about substitutions or in explaining the effects of continued use of diets of one form or another. This is especially important with members who have additional health problems as well. The nurse also has knowledge of illnesses that have as a symptom, obesity. The nurse in these groups can perform an important liaison function between other health services and these groups. Nurses may be in a position to refer clients to these groups or to assist members in getting additional help outside the group for physical or emotional problems.

Colostomy, laryngectomy, and other patient clubs or groups

A final example of self-help groups discussed in this text is the group whose members suffer some physical defect or disability such as that resulting from an accident or a necessary surgical correction. Instances of these kinds of groups may be colostomy or laryngectomy clubs. Frequently these groups extend services both in the hospital and in the community at large. They typically contact prospective members while these members are still in the hospital. The nurse is often instrumental in introducing patients to these groups or clubs.

The problems of members in these groups reflect problems caused by their recent handicap or disability. Sometimes members have not anticipated this disability or were not sufficiently prepared emotionally. They may suffer a variety of concerns related to the changes in their body—their ability to meet job responsibilities, their attractiveness to others, and their ability to accept or take care of their own impairment. Immediate postoperative reactions, for example, often involve an unrealistic perception of one's impairment as well as a frank rejection of the specific part of the body involved. Some patients do not even want to look at that part of their body "made ugly." These patients doubt whether they will be able to adapt and lack practical information about how they will be able to confront everyday life situations outside the hospital.

Visits from members of these clubs or groups while patients are still in the hospital are likely to increase the possibility that these patients will become members also. During and following their hospitalization, patients can gain support and understanding as well as useful information from these clubs or groups. The support and understanding that members receive in these groups are important ingredients both for those members who are giving and for those who are receiving. Members who receive support and understanding from others in the group are able to confront more courageously the frustrations and restrictions they experience with their disability. The giving of support and understanding enables members to experience feelings of self-worth partly taken away by their disability. This exchange tends to bind members together in a cooperative and self-enhancing relationship not possible with others who have not suffered from this disability.

Added impetus to adapt is provided through the role models in the group. The newcomer to the group has often lost hope that he will resume that function of himself affected by his disability, for example, his ability to make himself understood in the case of the laryngectomy patient. Still he is able to see that others have invented ways of adapting—of acquiring new skills and of masking their defect. Role models give members an alternative view of what their life may become, in spite of the disability.

Self-help groups or clubs for these patients can also provide members with a wealth of practical information about how to care for the disability, how to improve family relationships, or how to cope with the disability on the job or in social situations. Much of the information is that gained by the experience of others and therefore is usually practical and extremely relevant.

A final benefit of these groups to their members may be in terms of financial aid or provision of necessary equipment required because of the disability. These groups on occasion have been known to deter the costs of equipment or instruct members about getting aid from other sources, for example, foundations.

The role of nurses as resource persons in these groups can be extremely helpful. Nurses in the hospital and in the community have professional knowledge and skills related to members' disabilities; also, they often have information about how members can receive financial aid. Their actual knowledge regarding the care and limitations of members' disabilities, as well as their interventions, and the ability to implement this knowledge in the home setting could be quite helpful to members. If members need additional care, such as extra counseling or home health aides, they may provide for it or refer members to the appropriate agencies. They may also assist the group in determining who needs extra help. Essentially, then, they would not usurp the efforts of the group or club but would attempt to complement these efforts.

Other self-help and self-help health groups

The proliferation and growth in numbers and kinds of self-help endeavors assures us that this trend is becoming more predominant. The numbers of self-help health groups, especially women's clinics, have presented professionals an interesting challenge. Obviously the gap between professional services and meeting community needs, as the public defines them, is bridged by these clinics. Yet we have little documentation as to the quality of service members are receiving at reduced rates.

Groups (for example, Recovery, Inc.) and other organizations for psychiatric patients reduce patients' feelings of shame and isolation. "Dealing with fears" groups (for example, groups for phobic personalities) establish a basic "hot-line" system whereby patients can call one another in the middle of a crisis. Patients no longer feel they are alone with an irrational experience and benefit from the empathy shared in the group. Symptoms are the basis for embarrassment for many of the clients I have worked with. Patients are both afraid of their symptoms and fearful of rejection by "normal" people around them; the continued support from others who share and experience similar concern can sometimes make the difference in motivation to stay outside the walls of the institution.

Organizations of Parents Anonymous and Parents Without Partners, two quite different self-help groups, are also expanding. Parents Anonymous enables parents to control their child-abusive gestures; Parents Without Partners assists parents to gain support, advice, and coping strategies from other people who face the difficulties of single parenthood. The experiential basis—if you have or have had the problem, then you are a source of assitance to others—is still the number one ingredient in self-help groups and something professional services cannot adequately duplicate.

REFERENCES

1. Goffman, E.: Asylums, Garden City, N.Y., 1961, Doubleday & Co.
2. Marram, G.: Lectures for "basic psychiatric nursing," continuing education in nursing, San Francisco, 1967, University of California Medical Center.
3. Marram, G.: Substitution of Alcoholics Anonymous for "the bottle." Paper presented to Daniel Adelson, Ph.D, for a course in group dynamics, San Francisco, 1964. University of California Medical Center.
4. Verden, P., and Shatterly, D.: Alcoholism research. In Golden Gate Group Psychotherapy Society: Summaries of papers, San Francisco, 1969, The Society.
5. Wagonfeld, S., and Wolowitz, H. M.: Obesity and the self-help group: a look at TOPS, Am. J. Psychiatry **125:**249-252, 1968.

SUGGESTED READINGS
Introduction

Brembalo, J., and Young, D.: The self-help phenomena, Am. J. Nurs. **73:**1588-1591, 1973.

Gould, E., Garriques, C., and Schirkowitz, K.: Interaction in hospitalized patient-led and staff-led psychotherapy groups, Am. J. Psychother. **29:**383-390, 1975.

J. Appl. Behav. Sci. (entire issue) vol. 12, no. 3, 1976.

Katz, A., and Bender, E.: The strength in us: self-help groups in the modern world, New York, 1976, Franklin Watts.

Jerlson, J.: Self-help groups, Soc. Work **20:**144-145, 1975.

Silverman, P.: Mutual help: A guide for mental health workers, Washington, D.C., 1976, Government Printing Office.

Informal subgroups in institutions

McCorkle, L., and Korn, R.: Resocialization within walls, Ann. Sociol. **293:**88, 1954.

Stanton, A., and Schwartz, M.: The mental hospital, New York, 1954, Basic Books, Inc., Publishers.

Steinman, R., and Traunstein, D.: Redefining deviance: the self-help challenge to the human services, J. Appl. Behav. Sci. **12:**347-363, 1976.

Alcoholics Anonymous and its auxiliary groups

Alcoholics Anonymous: Alcoholics Anonymous, New York, 1937, A. A. World Services.

Alcoholics Anonymous: Twelve steps and twelve traditions, New York, 1952, A. A. World Services.

Berman, K. K.: Multiple conjoint family groups in the treatment of alcoholics, J. Med. Soc. N.J. **65:**6-8, 1968.

Burton, G.: An alcoholic in the family, Nurs. Outlook **12:**30-33, 1964.

Canter, F. M.: A self-help project with hospitalized alcoholics, Int. J. Group Psychother. **19:** 16-28, 1969.

Carroll, J. L., and Fuller, G. B.: The self and ideal-self concept of the alcoholic as influenced by length of sobriety and participation in Alcoholics Anonymous, J. Clin. Psychol. **25:**363-364, 1969.

Fox, R.: Group psychotherapy with alcoholics. In Rosenbaum, M., and Berger, M., editors: Group psychotherapy and group function, ed. 2, New York, 1975, Basic Books, Inc., Publishers.

Gillespie, C.: Nurses help combat alcoholism, Am. J. Nurs. **69:**1936-1941, 1969.

Killins, C. G., and Wells, C. L.: Group therapy of alcoholics, Curr. Psychiatr. Ther. **7:**174-178, 1967.

Mascarenhas, E., Hanrahan, F. R., and Plucinsky, J. J.: Rosary Hall—an AA-oriented hospital alcoholic care unit, Ohio State Med. J. **66:**812-814, 1970.

McCarthy, R. G.: Alcoholism, Am. J. Nurs. **59:**203-205, 1959.

Rubington, E.: The halfway house for the alcoholic, Ment. Hyg. **51:**552-560, 1967.
Ryberg, P. E.: A combined hospital setting and AA in the treatment of alcoholics, Behav. Neuropsychiatry **1:**19-21, 1969.
Wolff, K.: Group therapy for alcoholics, Ment. Hyg. **51:**549-551, 1967.

Synanon groups and other organizations for the drug addict
Casriel, D.: So fair a house: the story of synanon, Englewood Cliffs, N.J., 1963, Prentice-Hall.
LaLancette, T.: The nurse and the narcotic addict, J. Psychiatr. Nurs. **1:**29-33, 1963.
Rosenthal, M. S., and Biase, D. J.: Phoenix houses: therapeutic communities for drug addicts, Hosp. Community Psychiatry **20:**26-30, 1969.
Yablonsky, L.: Synanon: the tunnel back, New York, 1965, The Macmillan Co.

TOPS, Weight Watchers, and other weight-reducing groups
Candler, M. L.: Do we eat to live? J. Am. Med. Wom. Assoc. **23:**805-808, 1968.
Flack, R., and Grayer, E.: A conscious-raising group for obese women, Soc. Work **20:**484-487, 1975.
Kopelke, C.: Group education to reduce overweight, Am. J. Nurs. **75:**1993-1995, 1975.

Other self-help and self-help health groups
Comstock, B., and McDermott, M.: Group therapy for patients who attempt suicide, Int. J. Group Psychother. **25:**41-49, 1975.
Copeland, H., and Resnik, E.: The Tuesday evening club: using community resources to treat chronically ill patients, Hosp. Community Psychiatry **26:**227-230, 1975.
Grosz, H.: Recovery, Inc., Chicago, 1972, Recovery, Inc.
Marieskind, H., and Ehrenreich, B.: Toward socialist medicine: the women's health movement, Soc. Policy **6:**34-42, 1975.

CHAPTER 4

Growth and self-actualization groups

Introduction

Growth and self-actualization groups have gained increasing popularity since their inception in the late 1940s. Basically they originated as techniques employed by educators, and to a larger extent by social psychologists, to study and enhance human growth and development. Their history and development, use, and goals differ from those of any other category of group work, and only recently have they been utilized by disciplines whose task traditionally has been treatment. Their association with psychiatry and psychotherapy is probably more a result of the relaxation of territorial domains between these disciplines and of the tendency for psychiatry to shift to a focus on health, than it is a result of any conscious attempt to incorporate these types of groups as additional techniques in psychotherapy.

Growth and self-actualization groups began in an atmosphere of concern generated by social scientists for finding a method of teaching participatory democracy. The methodology employed in the 1940s stressed task-oriented group functioning, problem solving, and group process.[6] Chiefly the task, as perceived by social scientists, was to design educational processes to help learners incorporate values of democracy into their own processes of personal and collective decision making and problem solving.[2] Although there was some shift in the 1950s and 1960s from educative goals, for example, toward democratic participation in collective decision making and problem solving, these earlier concerns are reflected in a number of growth and self-actualization groups today. Emphases on experimentation, feedback, and collective deliberation permeate the operations of many of these groups. A democratically free and permissive atmosphere, where suppression and authoritarian leadership are prohibited, characterizes the nature of most growth and self-actualization groups today.

The emphasis on educative goals versus solely the more therapeutic goals of self-awareness, self-discovery, and self-actualization is still felt in these groups. Many groups, including marathon and encounter groups, present a certain amount of theoretical material with regard to perception, group process, and individual functioning. Likewise, many groups aim at increasing members' ability to achieve greater skill and knowledge in order to be more effective on the job. An emphasis on "take-home" knowledge and an intellectual basis for understanding their experiences are remnants of the earlier focus on educative goals per se. The degree to which groups today encourage a purely cognitive experience as opposed to an affective one is, however, likely to vary greatly.

Since their beginnings, essentially as group dynamics groups and sensitivity training groups, in the establishment of the National Training Laboratory (NTL), these groups have expanded to include various encounter, marathon, body movement, and creativity groups. A variety of organizations and institutions are known to sponsor these groups. Schools, churches, colleges, civic groups, businesses, and industries are a few of the organizations that arrange for these group experiences. These groups may be held within the institutions, for example, in a separate classroom in a school, or may be held outside the institution on a retreat in a nearby seaside resort or mountain lodge. It is not unusual to see a variety of persons participating in a single group experience; groups might be made up of lawyers, clergy, teachers, politicians, policemen, social workers, and nurses. Some groups may deal more exclusively with one professional group, as a management group whose members work together or a nurse supervisor and her staff. In addition to being made up of a variety of persons in different combinations, these groups are also led by a variety of professional and lay persons. Professionals—nurses, businessmen, psychologists, the clergy, educators, administrators—frequently lead such groups. Yet it is not uncommon to see someone in the community at large who has had no college or professional education leading these groups. The latter frequently occurs when special social issues—race relations, the generation gap, police-community relations—take on a secondary focus of the group.

Essentially the focus of growth and self-actualization groups is primarily one related to the education and self-enhancement of individuals in the group setting. Although the shift from purely educative to educative and therapeutic goals can be interpreted as a shift toward group psychotherapy, the focus of growth and self-actualization groups should not be confused with the focus of group psychotherapy or other groups. Growth and self-actualization groups do not seek insight for personality reconstruction; rather they focus on education and self-enhancement. New facets of one's behavior and feelings are realized in these groups, but the basic personality structure of persons remains unchanged. In growth and self-actualization groups, data about present behavior—the here and now in the group—is utilized rather than delving into genetic causes. Likewise, they deal with conscious behavior rather than with unconscious motivations.[2] Unlike members of group psychotherapy groups, members of growth and self-actualization groups are not asking for alleviation of symptoms caused by a neurotic or psychotic condition. They are primarily healthy individuals who want to improve their knowledge and skill in working or relating to others and who benefit from cognitive changes provided by the group experience.[9]

The focus of these groups is also different from that of therapeutic groups and self-help groups. Growth and self-actualization groups neither focus exclusively on problem solving nor operate to repress destructive impulses. Unlike typical therapeutic group situations, there is usually no specific situational or developmental crisis to which members are responding. These groups are not concerned with preventing some further psychological deterioration. Although socialization and support are important in these groups, they take on far less importance than in self-help groups. Support in some instances is thought to prevent the achievement of further self-discovery, although it is necessary to some extent if members are to develop a sense of security about testing new ways of reacting in the group. Self-enhancement and self-discovery, as viewed by many leaders of growth and self-actualization groups, require an atmosphere where current presentation of self is not taken for granted and allowed to crystallize in a new interpersonal situation. Self-enhancement in self-help groups, on the other hand, may only be permitted to the extent that it is circumscribed, for example, in so far as it facilitates the alcoholic's ability to relinquish his former drinking behavior.

The benefits that members receive from participating in growth and self-actualization groups are not always easily identifiable and easily documented. Many participants report vague feelings of elation, "freedom," or interpersonal satisfaction that are difficult to pinpoint or specify exactly but that seem to relate to some positive affective quality that they associate with the group itself, with certain others in the group, as the leader, or with their own participation and personal achievements in the group.

It is likely that to some degree this affective response relates to the phenomena observed by Burke and Bennis[4] that members become increasingly satisfied with their perception of self. These behavioral theorists explain that members, essentially of T-groups, became more satisfied with their perception of self, that is, move their actual self-perception in the direction of their ideal. Fortune[6] noted that members quite often leave these groups reluctant to discuss their experience for fear that the good feeling about self will vanish. In an attempt to counter this mystique, some group leaders insist that the transformation of self experienced in the group is not a single event, but should be viewed as a step in an ongoing process of self-actualization.

A benefit closely linked with the positive affective experience members have in the group is that of freedom to express oneself in new ways. Standards and norms in these groups encourage the expression of feelings and impulses, at the same time providing the needed redirection for those feelings and drives not conducive to effective, long-range social functioning. Sometimes these groups employ special techniques, for example, "warm-up" exercises, demonstrations, role playing, psychodrama, meditation, and yoga to enhance the expression of feelings and to encourage members to relate to one another in uncustomary and less stereotyped fashion. These opportunities for experiencing others in new ways and expressing oneself in new and sometimes unorthodox ways are both severly criticized and at the same time found to be quite personally satisfying to members. Leaders will often encourage members to participate as freely as possible and in whatever way they can. Such behavior as touching, holding, embracing, and fist fighting can at first be quite distressing to members. Still in time they are able to regard this behavior in a different light and utilize the opportunity comfortably. Members usually gain increased awareness of their inhibitions and possible bases for them. In addition, members discover that they can be themselves—do what they feel and say what they think—without disastrous effects.

Freedom of expression in these groups allows members to become more aware, not only of their inhibitions but also of their hidden capacities to relate to others. Members are encouraged to leave behind such usual symbols as formal attire and titles, objects that in the past have enabled them to relate comfortably. They gain increased awareness of how others perceive them without former disguises; quite often members are surprised and delighted that they can be liked and respected without these crutches. In addition it impels them to utilize certain personality attributes, for example, an ability to support others or to give feedback, in substitution for relating through roles or title.

Improvement of such interpersonal skills as relationships on the job is an anticipated and primary benefit promised by growth and self-actualization groups. Although change in this area is not an expressed benefit in some cases, it is implied in the goals of almost every group of this nature. Positive changes in interpersonal relations on the job and at home is the major goal of human relations and sensitivity training groups. Many professional training programs will offer such group experiences to enhance members' abilities to deal with clients or persons in authority.

Although changes in one's ability to relate to others is expected, changes of a wide variety often occur in such groups. These include perceptual, cognitive, and attitudinal changes, all of which influence members' behavioral changes. Consciousness-raising groups affect members' attitudes about key personal features that may have been denied recognition and appreciation by the individual. Sex, race, ethnic, and age characteristics become a focus for greater personal understanding and awareness.

The selection of individuals for these groups should be guided by the overall goals of the group and by the fact that group members are basically healthy individuals who wish to improve their knowledge and skill in relating to others or who seek further self-enhancement.

These groups are not appropriate for persons with frank psychotic or neurotic manifestations. They are not intended for sick people but for the "normal"—those who have good coping skills and who can readily learn from experience. A person is selected for therapy because he lacks ego skills and does not learn from his everyday life experiences.[7]

The reasons motivating many "normal" persons to seek out such a group experience are, of course, numerous. They may include certain expectations for therapy. More frequently, however, members join such a group to learn new techniques to use with people, to learn how to lead these groups themselves, or merely to get a quick emotional "kick."

One concern of many leaders is that members who elect to participate for the wrong reasons will have a potentially hazardous experience. Members, for example, who look for an escape, for therapy, or for marriage counseling in these groups can become dependent on them without realizing that such experiences are not appropriate for their needs. Most leaders believe it is extremely difficult to screen participants, and as Wyatt[11] explains, it is important that members be informed ahead of time of the appropriateness of the group for the needs members seek to meet. Participants often do not have enough information about what a group experience will offer or will be prior to participating. Some groups prohibit members who are currently in therapy.

In addition to being inappropriate for persons needing therapy, these groups are also inappropriate for individuals facing immediate developmental or situational crises. They are not concerned with preventing further psychological deterioration. Many of the growth and actualization groups are, however, being employed with young people in the schools. There is not sufficient evidence that such groups with normal children are harmful or, for that matter, beneficial. Parents have expressed concern that these groups are not appropriate in the school curriculum and can be harmful.

Lastly, as was pointed out earlier, these groups are also inappropriate for persons with special problems such as alcoholism and drug addiction. The goal of growth groups to open up a variety of new behaviors to members is not altogether in keeping with these persons' needs to suppress behavioral patterns. In the above instances, with regard to developmental and situational crises, as well as with special problems, therapeutic groups and self-help groups, respectively, are far more appropriate.

The preparation and role of the leader or trainer in such groups is usually quite varied. The majority of leaders have had some professional training; the type of training and its extensiveness are likely to be dissimilar. Some leaders—clergy, businessmen, nurses—may have had special orientations to human relations development, for example, the training at the National Training Laboratories (NTL), Boston University, or Escalen Institute. A larger number of persons become trainers through more informal processes. Some may have had group experiences with persons who have gone to the NTL. Still others may have had special courses in human relations and have coled with more experienced leaders. According to Wyatt,[11] informal processes usually include participating as a member in a group, observing and discussing experiences with others, being a coleader with another more experienced leader, and taking formal courses in human relations, humanistic psychology, change, organizational development, or Gestalt therapy.

In addition to the large number of professional persons leading these groups, some leaders have had no college education or specific professional orientation. Still they may have experienced a group themselves and become interested in leading these groups. Quite frequently those persons who also have special life experiences, for example, experience with race relations, will colead with a leader who has been prepared specifically to lead growth groups.

Most leaders today believe it is important that they have a background and experience somewhat related to the needs of the members in addition to having informal or formal education and training specific to leading these groups. A nurse who wishes to lead these groups may be especially useful to a group that consists of nurses or other health professionals.

Included in the nurse's formal learning experiences may be any combination of the following: membership in groups and leading and coleading experiences in these groups. Experience as a leader with supervision is of tremendous help to the neophyte and may aid nurses in becoming more aware of (1) their motivation for leading these groups, (2) their capacities and limitations as a leader, and (3) how others view their participation in the group. Of equal importance is the formal theoretical preparation nurses receive prior to or during their participation in the group. A background in group dynamics, group process, planned change, group leadership, and individual growth and development is necessary. Additional preparation to aid nurses in differentiating "normal" and "abnormal" behavior in the group and to provide them with special techniques such as role playing may be helpful. I have led several sensitivity training groups and have had extensive preparation in group psychotherapy as well. Whereas such preparation does seem to enhance one's ease in leading these groups, one's knowledge of techniques, and one's ability to monitor members' reactions to the group experience, it would seem that such preparation is not altogether essential to nurses who wish to lead or colead growth groups.

What is becoming more and more evident with respect to the preparation of good leaders is that members or clients need to be aware of what preparation they can expect from a leader and what additional professional or personal qualities are needed if the leader is to be appropriate for them. In the last few years many persons have assumed leadership positions after limited experience and in light of a limited talent to be sensitive toward others. Because of this, clients and client agencies will be more cautious, or should be, about the persons they select to lead such groups. Nurses, like other professional and lay persons who want to lead these groups, should not expect that they will be able to convince clients to accept their limited experience and preparation as adequate credentials.

Group dynamics groups

Group dynamics groups have been employed widely during the past two decades to improve the skill and knowledge of members with regard to group decision making and group process. The techniques utilized in these groups such as role playing, buzz sessions, and observation and assessment of group movement are utilized in a number of growth and self-actualization groups, especially sensitivity training programs designed to improve the skill of members in human relations and management.[5] Different from most T-groups, as well as from marathons and encounters, group dynamics groups emphasize the cognitive acquisition of knowledge about groups, group decision making, and group process.

The term *group dynamics* itself has been used to refer not only to a form of group experience and to a set of techniques but also to a sort of political ideology and a field of inquiry. Cartwright and Zander[5] have specified that group dynamics as a political ideology is concerned with the way groups should be organized and managed. As an ideology it emphasizes the importance of democratic leadership, the participation of members in decisions, and the benefits both to society and the individual to be obtained through cooperative activities in groups. Finally, as a field of inquiry, group dynamics is concerned with achieving knowledge about the nature of groups, the laws of their development, and their relationships with individuals, groups, and large institutions. What is sometimes quite evident in group dynamics groups is that group dynamics as an ideology and system of inquiry permeates the group's activities and goals and members' interaction within the group.

The concerns of members in group dynamics groups are sometimes quite clearly aligned with the ideology and system of inquiry. Those who sponsor group dynamics groups, for example, management divisions or large industries and business firms, are often concerned with employing "democratic" leadership and collective decision making on the job. Managers are encouraged to participate in group dynamics groups and workshops in order to be familiar with and incorporate these elements in their relations with subordinates. Professional education and training, such as nursing programs, may also utilize these groups for similar reasons. In the preparation of team leaders or administrators, nursing schools and hospitals often persuade nurses to participate in these groups in order to get them to use democratic leadership techniques in the management of their nursing staff.

Another significant group of individuals who participate in group dynamics groups are those who, as a part of their training for a special field, need to learn about the nature of groups and the laws that govern group development and group process. This is a group that intends to be involved extensively in group work, group psychotherapy, or therapeutic group work, for instance. Community mental health nursing programs which anticipate that their graduates will be utilizing a number of group approaches with clients may require students to have a group dynamics group experience, as well as leadership experience in other types of groups. This requirement is intended to provide students with a basic foundation of experience and knowledge related to group process, group development, and individual behavior in groups.

Group dynamics groups have been known to produce a number of benefits with regard to the operation of existing groups, but also with regard to individual members' acquisition of new knowledge and skill about groups. Among the various cognitive changes that have been noted in members are (1) increased awareness of group movement and phases of group development, (2) increased understanding of group process and how individual roles interact in the group, (3) increased understanding of the limitations and benefits of democratic leadership and collective decision making, and (4) a better understanding of the meaning of leadership and leader activities in a group.

Beyond the important cognitive changes that occur with members, certain attitudinal and behavioral changes occur that improve their functioning in the group and in other groups in which they are involved. It is not uncommon for a team of manager and salesmen or supervisor and nurses, for example, to exercise more effective decision making or more democratic leadership after the team has been exposed to a group dynamics group or workshop. Concomitant with their change in ability to work together are certain attitudinal changes, such as a belief that delegation of authority can be efficient and effective and a belief that leadership should be shared with respect to members' areas of expertise (professional and personal expertise), as well as a belief that democratic leadership is not always feasible or desirable in cases of collective decision making.

The role of the nurse as a leader in these groups has traditionally been one of coleadership with another professional, for example, a social psychologist or educator. Some nurses have assumed full leadership of these groups with outside supervision by psychologists. Nurses who do choose to lead and colead in these groups must have basically two types of knowledge: (1) knowledge of the specific decision-making and organizational problems members confront on a day-to-day basis with their jobs and (2) extensive knowledge of groups, group process, groups within larger institutions and organizations, group development, and leadership development. In addition they must share the ideology that is put forth by a group dynamics orientation, that is, a commitment and belief in collective decision making and democratic principles. More concretely they must have faith that the group can solve its problems without their authoritative intervention. On the other hand, they must know the limits of the group to employ democratic action at any one time and must be prepared to assume a more active role at different points in the group. The problems that most leaders or facilitators experience are those related to knowing how active or passive they should be at different times in the group. Trust in the group, yet a sensitivity about when to intervene, is essential to the nurse. Supervision of their own role in the group by an experienced group leader may enable leaders to become more aware of how their role can either enhance or disrupt the group in its attempts to employ democratic principles and at the same time learn about group development and group process. Sometimes their interventions are based more on unrealistic concerns about what will happen to the members if they avoid intervening—unrealistic concerns that may have arisen out of their own previous group experiences. Supervision of their role by an experienced group leader will often bring this to their awareness, and they will have an opportunity to change their approach if it is necessary.

Sensitivity training or T-groups

Closely akin to group dynamics groups is the sensitivity or T-group. Essentially most group dynamics groups are thought to be sensitivity training groups. These two groups are differentiated here in an attempt to clarify differences in the emphases in these groups.

Sensitivity training groups frequently use techniques such as role playing employed by group dynamics groups. Also, T-groups do aim for certain cognitive changes in members, for example, the acquisition of knowledge related to collective decision making and group process.

T-groups, however, emphasize to a greater extent cognitive changes with reference to awareness of self and others as opposed to change toward acquiring greater knowledge. These groups approach management problems more directly by encouraging subordinates and supraordinates to become aware of the feelings of each other and of the effect of their own behavior on others. Essentially the chief aim is increased sensitivity toward others in the group. Increased knowledge of group development can, however, be one outcome of increased sensitivity in these groups and is espoused by those who developed the sensitivity group. (See Bradford, Gibb, and Benne.[2])

The early proponents of group dynamics groups recognized the very real difficulties in utilizing democratic processes in everyday life situations. They believed that operational definitions of democratic values were necessary if they were to be more relevant to conditions of contemporary living.[2] The practical task as they saw it was to design experiences that would help individuals to incorporate these values in a practical way—one such experience was seen to be the sensitivity training laboratory or unstructured group in which members can learn to function cooperatively while becoming more fully aware of themselves and others.

The term *T-group* or *sensitivity group* is now loosely used to include a wide range of laboratory approaches to affective learning. Persons who participate in each of these groups for the most part have much in common. One difference, however, is that persons who wish sensitivity group experience may desire less affective involvement than those who seek out marathon or encounter groups but desire more affective involvement than is experienced in the traditional forms of group dynamics groups.

Many individuals who participate in group dynamics groups at some point also have a sensitivity training experience. These individuals can be of the management or administrative type or of the student type. Managers and their subordinates who are experiencing collective decision-making problems also are likely to engage together in an experience where they can learn about one another and experiment with new ways of relating. T-groups and sensitivity groups with respect to students in professional education are utilized basically for the same reasons: to provide them with a more effective basis of learning about others in an unstructured group setting.

Yeaworth[12] has adequately specified four essential designs describing the makeup of these groups: *Stranger T-groups* involve persons from different walks of life, for example, the clergy, businessmen, teachers, and lawyers in one group. *Common experience T-groups* have participants who share common occupations, professional identities, or interests. *Working T-groups* involve teams of persons, as teams of salesmen from a company or nurse supervisors and their staff. These members already have established relationships on the job. A fourth type of T-group is what Yeaworth refers to as a *merger intergroup*. This type of group has as its objective the reduction of conflict resulting from the merger of different groups within organizations.

T-groups are the major laboratory experiences sponsored by the National Training Laboratories. The focus is on learning rather than on therapy. Members have, as it is conceived, in their day-to-day interaction with others grown accustomed to the tact, courtesy, and veiled expression of feelings that reduce effective communication and that do not award them the feedback they need and desire. Likewise, as is true on the job, much of members' behavior and interaction with others is a function of the roles and positions they occupy. The amount of personal feedback about oneself as a person is greatly reduced. Also, feedback persons do get from intimate, unstructured conversations is limited. According to Yeaworth,[12] in our society people are not receptive to nor appreciative of any type of feedback. Positive feedback may be interpreted as ingratiation or meaningless, and negative feedback as undesirable and cruel. With increasing industrialization, explains Yeaworth, people have abandoned ties to a single all-encompassing group. T-groups offer people in industry, professionals who work in such an atmosphere, and students who are the by-products of an industrialized age an alternative to the types of learning and feedback experiences they receive in the society at large and on the job. T-groups give one a chance to associate with others who have similar concerns, to drop one's customary role, to reveal facets of the self that have become obscured in the rush of everyday living and in the responses to roles, and to give and receive negative and positive feedback. Often, one can try out in the group new behaviors or the expression of masked feelings without the risk that would be involved otherwise, that is, in places where it was not understood that members should experiment with new ways of relating to each other.

The benefits of T-groups, although varied, may best be described as increased self-awareness, intellectual understanding of group functioning, and awareness of others. Unlike many other educational practices, T-groups achieve these benefits through experience-based learning in unstructured group experiences. Increased self-awareness is furthered by the fact that members enter these groups and are dispossessed of roles and such other self-defining equipment as title, position, and uniform. They experience increased anxiety about themselves as individuals without predefined identities; this causes personal stress but, in turn, allows members to come in touch with "the real me."[8] Along with the experience of getting to know oneself is that of gaining increased knowledge of how a group functions.

Quite often in T-group settings the leader will purposively redirect the experience from a tense, emotional self-awareness to an intellectual discussion of: "what is happening in the group right now," or "let's examine (and put into perspective) some of the phases that we as a group have gone through up to now." The shift, with the aid of the leader, from an intense emotional experience to a purely intellectual exercise is intended not only to relieve anxiety of members in the group but also to encourage the intellectual awareness of members about group functioning and group process. The incorporation of an intellectual grasp of group movement and group dynamics groups, although it is characteristically a remnant of group dynamics groups, if often utilized in T-groups. The extent to which the group will entertain intellectual exercises of this nature, when it does, and the emphasis placed on such learning depends on many things, including the philosophy of the agency or institution sponsoring the group and the preference and skill of the T-group trainer or leader.

Not totally distinct, but of value to members, is the increased awareness about others in the group. Quite often members, especially in management positions, enter these groups hoping to be able to understand and "get along with" their subordinates, peers, and supervisors. Their difficulties stem from a lack of sensitivity about the needs, fears, and concerns of others. Whether because they have intentionally desensitized themselves or whether because they have never been equipped to empathize with others, these members benefit greatly from opportunities to listen to and get feedback from other members in the group under intense emotional conditions.

Increased awareness of self and others, as well as increased intellectual awareness of group functioning in T-groups, has been known to carry over to members' relations on the job, in social situations, and with family members. Unfortunately systematic data about the long-term benefits or effects of T-groups is lacking. The nature of the benefits and effects is also not clearly understood. Still the National Training Laboratories, as well as other organizations that sponsor T-groups, do note that up to two-thirds of the participants increase their skills in interpersonal relationships after a T-group experience of some kind.[10]

The role of a nurse as a trainer or leader of T-groups differs little from that of any other trainer. More specifically, trainers can be viewed as "facilitators" of group process and member interaction who make it possible for T-groups to achieve their aims for increased awareness and sensitivity. The leader can assume a role conceived of as passive, at which time a comaraderie in the group is heightened to deemphasize former expectations about leaders and persons in authority. The leader can also assume an active role, described as being a didactic, authoritative position, at which time concrete information about group process and group functioning is presented. One very necessary skill of the leader is a sense of timing with regard to when a passive or more active role is required.

The role of the T-group leader in most cases, and in slight contrast with that of the group dynamics group leader, can be conceived of as a "nonleader" role. By not participating in the usual way, that is, in the way that members would expect any person in authority to participate, the leader facilitates a situation in which leadership behavior from the group members is necessary to solve group problems, for example, to formulate group goals. A lack of participation in the traditional manner causes members increased stress but at the same time brings to members' awareness the mechanisms of group problem solving and individual functioning in the group.

Most sensitivity trainers feel that making their role a psychotherapeutic one in terms of focusing on motivations for individual behavior, the unconscious, and transference relationships that develop in the group is beyond the bounds of a trainer's role. Still others utilize techniques to get members involved in the group, deeper, faster and on more than the here-and-now level. Whereas these techniques can be useful in seeking group involvement and early cohesiveness, the trainer does well to remember that one goal of the trainer is to encourage group members' solutions of group problems; the problem of lack of group member involvement is a problem the members must solve. Introjecting techniques for members does not allow them to come to a solution on their own. In addition the problem of involvement may be obscured and never realized by the group. Trainers do differ, however, with respect to what they feel is most important for members to achieve through the group experience. Those who aim at more awareness and exchange based on self-discovery may utilize techniques of this kind, whereas those who stress learning about group process and group problem solving will most likely utilize techniques to get deeper, faster to a lesser extent.

A number of skills have been identified as essential to the trainer or leader of T-groups, ranging from the possession of intuition, to a formal knowledge of groups and individual behavior, to an ability to employ techniques. Blake[1] and others have noted that the following may be necessary: (1) to identify the reason for behavior in the group, (2) to examine the subjective feelings of group members, (3) to become aware of assumptions on which the group is approaching a problem or task, and (4) to understand how membership roles and functions are being executed in the group. Blake sees the skills of the trainer to be different from those of the group psychotherapist; he emphasizes the ability of the trainer to help members become participant-observers with respect to the evaluation of what is going on in the group. Members then are not primarily dependent on the trainer's analysis.

The National Training Laboratories as well as trainers themselves recommend that leaders be emotionally well-adjusted individuals, as well as experienced and sensitive teachers of group dynamics. The emotional stability felt to be essential in trainers is most often linked with the trainer's ability to prevent the development of emotional breakdowns in members. Some trainers refer to this capacity as a "gut" feeling or intuition about the limitations and strengths of group members. Whereas this "gut" feeling does seem to be important, it should be noted that intuition is enhanced by the trainer's increased experience in groups, as well as by concrete knowledge of group processes. Obviously someone who is not "well adjusted" may not possess sensitivity to others because of his involvement with self or may not be able to view the group objectively enough to connect concrete thoughts with vague feelings he gets about what is helpful to the group members.

As a trainer in several sensitivity groups I noted that the skills and qualities mentioned here were essential to my success in leading these groups. In addition to these, however, supervision of one's leadership in a group is also helpful in keeping on top of members' concerns and needs, some of which may be overlooked during the session. Tape-recorded sessions that may be reviewed by the trainer and the supervisor are often quite helpful both in assessing the trainer's performance and in analyzing the interaction of members in the group.

Encounter groups

Perhaps the most obvious landmark in the shift of growth and self-actualization groups from purely educative goals to increased self-discovery via intense involvement with others in a group is the encounter group. Basically the encounter group is not totally dissimilar to the T-group. It is a group experience in which members can expect to become closer to their "authentic" selves, to leave masquerades behind, and to enjoy the uncensored interaction with others they are not allowed in their everyday life in an industrialized, depersonalized society.

Encounter groups do, however, differ from T-groups. Encounter groups focus on the individual group member's needs for greater understanding of self and self-discovery.[3] Unlike the sensitivity and group dynamics group, the encounter group is less likely to allow members to intellectualize about any part of their experience in the group. These groups essentially offer an experience beyond the shelter of focusing on the group or on others in the group. On occasion the encounter group has been likened to a religious experience. With the addition of the residential dimension—that is, when the group is a residential encounter group—the group's impact on individuals can be increased. Basically members in these groups are encouraged to level with each other about their feelings and their reactions to others. At the outset most participants have the intention of improving their interpersonal competence. This need is not totally unlike that of T-group participants. Still their need is more concerned with freeing the self from unnecessary social constraints in order to reach an authentic encounter with others. T-groups and group dynamics groups, per se, are not believed to enable members to meet these needs as much as encounter groups do. Part of the rationale for the encounter approach lies with the concern that the intellectualizing permitted in T-groups and group dynamics groups is a constraint that prohibits members from reacting to one another in an immediate and open manner. The idea of the encounter approach is conceived of as a need of members to disclose aspects of themselves usually kept hidden through the process of objectifying or intellectualizing about experiences.

The benefits of encounter groups for members are related to members' needs for increased interpersonal competence and authenticity. Being able to disclose hidden aspects of the self is thought to reduce the sense of aloneness that members experience in our industrialized, depersonalized society. As feelings of being "all alone" diminish, strong emotional bonds are likely to form between members in the group. These bonds occur particularly when the group members essentially live together, for example, for a weekend or two-week period in residential encounter groups. The security that generates from these close relationships with other members in turn aids members to become more authentic in their interaction with others in the group and to abandon former social or professional facades.

As participants become more involved with each other in the group, they become acutely aware of interpersonal problems that they have had with others, especially when intense feelings were generated. As they rediscover interpersonal problems, they are encouraged to work on them with others in the group. Quite often members realize that these problems form a life pattern. On occasion the special conditions of the group—the security, trust, feedback, and permissiveness—promote a breakthrough for them.

The emotional climate of the encounter group differs greatly from that of the outside world, and the reentry is often painful, even more so than for those who have participated in T-groups. Members yearn for the opportunity to extend the experience beyond the group and make the authenticity they were able to achieve in the group an integral part of their daily lives. The problem of articulating this experience with their everyday life experiences is noted by most members. Sometimes members realize that it was more the intense involvement as opposed to the interpersonal competence, per se, that they were seeking. All in all, however, members consider that they now have more alternative ways of behaving open to them. I have observed that this knowledge alone can have a tremendous impact on their relationships with others. They are usually less frustrated knowing that they chose to act as they did in light of a number of alternatives. Members interact with others in social, personal, and professional relationships with renewed energy and understanding of themselves. Likewise a change in their own attitudes may affect how others respond to them. For example, one member's ability to cry when he was hurt, instead of getting angry as he usually did, caused persons close to him to empathize with him instead of getting angry in return.

The role of the nurse or any professional leading encounter groups is a tremendously challenging one. Basically the nurse must possess a certain philosophy about members' and man's need for self-expression. I have found that most encounter group leaders believe that man needs to learn to better express his basic nature rather than to control or to direct impulses that are unsafe, destructive, or harmful to others.

As in the T-group, nurses who choose to lead the encounter group are more facilitators than leaders in the traditional sense. They may refuse to exert authority invested in them by the group. They may be passive with respect to the direction of the group and let topics go without intervention. They may give the group no clear task and avoid directing the group in discussion; they may even block some attempts at leadership. Nurses are more likely to do the latter when this leadership is intellectual in nature or is part of another facade the member is extending to prevent his relating to others on a feeling or more authentic level. Members' attempts to achieve leadership roles in the group may be viewed by the leader as attempts to set themselves apart from others, quite often in a "one-upmanship" manner.

The skills and knowledges essential to the nurse who leads encounter groups are not unlike those needed to lead other growth and self-actualization groups. Nurses must have a basic knowledge of group process and individual roles in groups. They must have a keen sense of timing with respect to utilizing techniques that arouse members to respond more spontaneously. Less concerned with the group's development, per se, and more with the outcome of the experience for each individual, they must be acutely aware of how members are manifesting themselves in the group and of how members might relinquish stereotyped patterns of relating to others.

Perhaps just as important is nurses' awareness of themselves. Nurses whose aim it is to help others to become more authentic must expect that they will be looked to as models; therefore they should have developed a certain level of authenticity themselves. Quite often leaders will talk with members about their own experiences with becoming more spontaneous and less defensive with others.

As with leadership roles in other groups, supervision by a more experienced leader can prove very helpful. This is especially so since nurses must be aware of their own problems of achieving authenticity with others and of how these problems influence the group.

Marathon and semimarathon groups

I have found that with the exception of the residential encounter group, marathon groups probably have a greater emotional impact on members than any other type of growth and self-actualization group. Like encounter groups, they produce a qualitatively different kind of experience from that usually expected with others in everyday life experiences. Basically the term *marathon* refers to how the group operates rather than to its unique scope or focus. Marathon groups per se may be likened to encounter groups and even some sensitivity groups. The aspect of continued, uninterrupted contact with members in the group, from 24 up to 48 hours, however, intensifies the experience greatly and increases the tendency for personal disclosure and temporary group solidarity. In turn the affect exchanged between members in the group is strongly emotional and usually intense.

Marathon groups serve a particular need for those persons unable or unwilling to devote two weeks (in an encounter group) or six months to a year (in a T-group) to developing greater self-awareness. They also enable persons with strong defenses against self-disclosure and interpersonal closeness an opportunity to break through this pattern and relate more openly to others. An experience that runs the entire weekend with breaks only for meals cannot help but intensify the group experience for members. Quite often, as noted by leaders of these groups, fatigue of members adds to the ability of the group to make a significant breakthrough in their former patterns of relating to others. Fatigue, as is noted in research on emotional disturbances, has a significant effect on individuals' ability to retain defensive mechanisms. The hope in the marathon group is that those mechanisms which are least dissatisfying or most disruptive of interpersonal interaction will be broken down, making room for new and more satisfying ways of responding to others.

The benefits of marathon groups, like those of encounter groups, are related to greater interpersonal competency and personal authenticity, rather than to the intellectual grasp of group process, group development, and group leadership. Marathon groups, and to a lesser extent, encounter groups, probably typify most the shift in growth and self-actualization groups from purely educative to more therapeutic purposes.

The intense contact with other members in the group that facilitates the diminished use of certain defense mechanisms in relating to others borders significantly on the goals of certain group therapy groups. Marathon groups differ, however, in two aspects from therapy groups. Members usually suffer no severe personality or emotional disturbance, and the personality reconstruction that occurs in these groups is often short lived. These groups do not intend to force personality reconstruction but merely want to give members the "taste" of different ways of being with others. Members are felt to possess sufficient amounts of ego strength to reinforce themselves in the use of new patterns of relating once given the "taste" of new patterns in the group.

Quite often, however, the ability of members to sustain new patterns of relating once outside the group is lacking. In a marathon, as well as in encounter groups, members' experiences seem to relate significantly to the fact that these groups create a kind of social-cultural island, isolated from the norms of the greater society. The tendency for members to relax their demands for interpersonal authenticity and personal disclosure "on the outside" is marked. This seems to be due in part to the fact that facades and emotional isolation in our society are more expedient and more acceptable elements in individuals' interactions with others.

Despite the fact that the effects of marathon groups are likely to be short lived, members' abilities to learn about themselves and others in the group and to adapt new ways of interacting are notable. The feedback members get from one another is likely to be more straightforward in these groups. Also, under conditions of intense and uninterrupted contact, members are more likely to trust the feedback they receive. The results of straight-forward feedback that is trusted by members open up communication and enable members to become highly sensitive to one another's feelings and needs. Outside the group, members are more likely to be keenly perceptive of different aspects of their own and others' communication.

The role of the nurse as a leader in marathon groups is similar to that in encounter groups. More specifically, in marathon groups, nurses must be able to facilitate members' quick, intense involvement with others, as well as trust in the group. Techniques are helpful and should be an integral part of the leader's activity in the group. Blindman's walk, for example, is a useful technique to encourage trust between members. (Techniques are taken up in Chapter 13.)

The nurse who leads an encounter group must be acutely aware of the emotional strengths and liabilities of members under conditions of intense interaction, where defense mechanisms are likely to be threatened. A knowledge of abnormal and normal behavior, skill in alleviating anxiety, and a capacity to make decisions about the use of marathons with various individuals is essential to the nurse. The knowledge and skills mentioned here should be useful to nurses in their selection of members for the group and will guide their interventions during the marathon session. The momentum of the group, once the session has started, is often difficult to interrupt: the nurse will find that careful scrutiny ahead of time about who should be included in the group is most important in the encounter group. Some leaders choose to interview each candidate personally before accepting them in the group.

Because marathon groups border more on therapy groups than do other self-actualization groups, some leaders recommend that leaders have extensive professional training such as in psychotherapy and group psychotherapy. Nurses who wish to lead marathon groups should have had graduate experience in group work, group psychotherapy, and abnormal behavior. Supervision, although it is not as feasible with these groups because marathons are uninterrupted group experiences, is advisable even on a post hoc basis. It is often the case that leaders of marathon groups will have a coleader who may serve as an "on the spot" check on the primary leader's activities in the group.

Other self-actualization formats

There is no doubt in my mind that growth, self-actualization, and consciousness-raising group formats are here to stay. Likewise, I hold a great deal of appreciation for the imagination of theorists and humanists to create new modes of stimulating our awareness and authenticity in relating to others. ARICA, biofeedback, ethnodrama, rolfing, group hypnotherapy, and EST (Erhard Seminar Training), to name a few, are further innovations in experiencing oneself that will be accompanied by still other self-actualization modes. The early use of group dynamics groups to learn human relations skills has taken a tremendous shift. Now we hold human relations training groups for psychiatric patients as well as the to-be-manager and college student. Self-directed, tape-directed, or leader-directed, one thing is clear: our ability to document the effects of these permutations has probably fallen behind our initiative to create new ways to deliver interpersonal effectiveness, "humanness," growth, and self-actualization.

REFERENCES

1. Blake, R. R.: Group training vs. group therapy, New York, 1958, Beacon House.
2. Bradford, L. P., Gibb, J. R., and Benne, K. D.: Two educational innovations. In Bradford, L., et al., editors: T-group theory and laboratory method, New York, 1964, John Wiley & Sons.
3. Bugental, J. F. T., and Haigh, G. V.: Psychology and retreats: frontier for experimentation. In Magee, R. J., editor: Call to adventure, Nashville, Tenn., 1968, Abingdon-Cokesbury.
4. Burke, R. L., and Bennis, W. G.: Changes in perception of self and others during human relations training, Hum. Rel. **14:**165-182, 1961.
5. Cartwright, D., and Zander, A., editors: Group dynamics—research and theory, ed. 4, New York, 1968, Harper & Row, Publishers.
6. Fortune, H. O.: The pros and cons of sensitivity training, Nurs. Outlook **18:**24-29, 1970.
7. Gottschalk, L. A., and Pattison, E. M.: Psychiatric perspectives on T-groups and the laboratory movement: an overview, Am. J. Psychiatry **126:**823-839, 1969.
8. Marram, G.: What is happening to nurses, Int. Nurs. Rev. **16:**320-328, 1969.
9. Miles, M. B.: The training group. In Bennis, W. G., et al., editors: The planning of change, New York, 1961, Holt, Rinehart & Winston.
10. National Training Laboratories Institute: News and reports, Washington D.C., 1969, The Institute, vol. 3, p. 2.
11. Wyatt, W. C.: Responsible use of sensitivity training, Nurs. Outlook **18:**39-40, 1970.
12. Yeaworth, R.: Learning through group experience, Nurs. Outlook **18:**29-32, 1970.

SUGGESTED READINGS
Introduction
Anderson, J.: Human relations training and group work, Soc. Work **20:**195-199, 1975.
Benne, K., et al.: The laboratory method of changing and learning: theory and application, Palo Alto, Calif., 1975, Science and Behavior Books.
Bradford, L. P., editor: Explorations in human relations training: an assessment of experiences 1947-1953, Washington, D.C., 1953, National Training Laboratory in Group Development, National Educational Association.
Johnson, D., and Johnson, F.: Joining together—group theory and group skills, Englewood Cliffs, N.J., 1975, Prentice-Hall.
Lewin, K.: Group decision and social change. In Proschanchy, H., and Siedenberg, B., editors: Basic studies in social psychology, New York, 1965, Holt, Rinehart & Winston.
Rosenberg, P. P., and Fuller, M. L.: Human relations seminar: a group work experimentation in nursing education, Ment. Hyg. **39:**406-432, 1955.
Shaffer, J., and Galinshy, M.: Models of group therapy and sensitivity training, Englewood Cliffs, N.J., 1974, Prentice-Hall.
Schein, E. H., and Bennis, W. G.: Personal and organizational change through group methods, New York, 1965, John Wiley & Sons.
Schutz, W. C.: Joy: expanding human awareness, New York, 1967, Grove Press.

Group dynamics groups
Benne, K. D.: Democratic ethics and human engineering. In Bennis, W. G. et. al., editors: The planning of change, New York, 1961, Holt, Rinehart & Winston.
Bonner, H.: Group dynamics—principles and applications, New York, 1959, The Ronald Press Co.
Cartwright, D., and Lippitt, R.: Group dynamics and the individual. In Bennis, W. G. et al., editors: The planning of change, New York, 1961, Holt, Rinehart & Winston.

Conte, W. R., and Waggoner, E. R.: The group dynamic approach to professional maturation, Am. J. Occup. Ther. **24:**343-346, 1970.
Knowles, M., and Knowles, H.: Introduction to group dynamics, New York, 1959, Association Press.

Sensitivity training or T-groups

Argyris, C.: T-groups for organizational effectiveness, Harvard Bus. Rev. **42:**60-74, 1964.
Birnbaum, M.: Sense about sensitivity training, Saturday Rev. **52:**82-83, 1969.
Blumberg, A., and Busche, M.: An inservice program in human relations, Nurs. Outlook **5:**703-705, 1957.
Cahn, M. W.: Where goes the T-group when it's over? Hum. Rel. Trng. News **13:**6, 1965.
Hollister, W. G.: Brainwashing vs. strengthening individuality, Hum. Rel. Trng. News **13:**1, 1969.
Lundgren, D., and Knight, D.: Trainer style and member attitudes toward trainers and group in T-groups, Small Group Behav. **8:**25-47, 1977.
Laschinsky, D., and Koch, U.: T-groups: origin, participants and goals, Psychother. Psychosom. **26:**39-48, 1975.
Reddy, W. B.: Sensitivity training or group psychotherapy: the need for adequate screening, Int. J. Group Psychother. **20:**336-349, 1970.
Smith, P.: Are there adverse effects of sensitivity training? J. Hum. Psychol. **15:**29-47, 1975.

Encounter groups

Egan, G.: Encounter: group processes for interpersonal growth, Belmont, Calif., 1970, Brooks/Cole Publishing Co.
Haas, K.: Growth encounter: a guide for groups, Chicago, 1975, Helson-Hall.
Peck, H. B.: Encounter and T-groups—the current use of the group for personal growth and development: introduction, Int. J. Group Psychother. **20:**263-266, 1970.
Rogers, C.: Carl Rogers groups on encounter, New York, 1970, Harper & Row, Publishers.
Shapiro, R., and Klein, R.: Perceptions of the leaders in an encounter group, Small Group Behav. **6:**238-248, 1975.
Watkins, J., et al.: Changes toward self-actualization, Small Group Behav. **6:**272-281, 1975.

Marathon and semimarathon groups

Chambers, W. M., and Ficek, D. E.: An evaluation of marathon counseling, Int. J. Group Psychother. **20:**372-379, 1970.
Dinges, N., and Weigel, R.: Evaluation of marathon groups and the group movement. In Suinn, R., and Weigel, R., editors: The innovative psychological therapies: critical and creative contributions, New York, 1975, Harper & Row, Publishers.
Jones, D., and Medvene, A.: Self-actualization effects of a marathon growth group, J. Couns. Psychol. **22:**39-43, 1975.
Myerhoff, H., Jacobs, A., and Holler, F.: Emotionality in marathon and traditional psychotherapy groups, Psychother. Theory Res. Prac. **7:**33-36, 1970.
Potheir, P. C.: Marathon encounter groups: rationale techniques and crucial issues, Perspect. Psychiatr. Care **8:**153-159, 1970.
Walker, M., and Holbert, W.: Perceived acceptance and helpfulness in a marathon group, Psychol. Rep. **27:**83-90, 1970.

Other self-actualization formats

Galassi, J., et al.: Assertive training: a one year follow-up, J. Couns. Psychol. **22:**451-452, 1975.
Osborn, S., and Harris, J.: Assertive training for women, Springfield, Ill., 1975, Charles C Thomas, Publisher.
Tounsend, R.: A comparison of biofeedback—mediated relaxation and group therapy in the treatment of chronic anxiety, Am. J. Psychiatry **132:**598-601, 1975.

CHAPTER 5

Reference groups

Introduction

Unlike all those groups discussed thus far, reference groups are not usually formulated for the specific purpose of achieving some therapeutic effect for members. Still it is quite clear that these groups do afford individuals certain benefits that relate to identity formation, self-concept, and self-esteem.

The term *reference group* in its most general sense is used to designate that kind of group, real or imaginary, whose position is used by an individual to view and judge objects or principles around him.[10] As a member of a reference group, the individual behaves with respect to a certain audience—the group. The reference group usually supports the values that the individual uses in evaluating his own conduct. A person's activities, then, can be said to depend on the real or anticipated reactions of the other people in his reference group.

Any individual can respond to various groups of referent others in this manner. Usually, however, there is one group that he utilizes more frequently than others in evaluating his behavior. Also, individuals may change reference groups or acquire new ones as they proceed through life and develop sustained contact with various persons around them. Reference groups are pervasive throughout an individual's life and play an important role in his concept of self.

Examples of reference groups and referent others that appear as a person ages may include any one or a combination of the following types of groups: religious, racial, ethnic, familial, and occupational reference groups. These groups are not ordinarily groups with which members will immediately acknowledge membership if they were asked directly to list the groups to which they belong. Membership in reference groups is somewhat different from membership in clubs or in organizations. Membership in many groups, in the traditional sense, encompasses a rather narrow conception of responsibility and obligation: "membership" in a reference group involves a vague, yet all-encompassing identification with others in the group. Essentially it is through the eyes of his referent others that a person establishes who he is and what he should do. NOTE: It is important to make the distinction clear here, that a number of groups which a person merely has membership in are not reference groups for him. A group of this kind could become a reference group to that individual if he had sustained contact with others in the group and continuously evaluated himself with reference to the values and standards of the group or group members. It has been suggested by many group theorists that long-term therapy or therapeutic groups become reference groups for members, and it is this fact that explains why group therapy succeeds.

Simply participating in a group, then, does not ordinarily indicate that the group is a reference group for members. According to Shibutani,[10] when individuals think, feel, and see things from the standpoint of the group, when the group helps them decide what goals are worth seeking and the manner in which one should pursue his aspirations, it may be conceived as a reference group for members. In part, then, whether a group is a reference group depends on the nature of the group, for example, whether it projects specific values and standards, and on the way that individuals react to these values and standards, that is, whether they allow them to direct their lives.

What seems pertinent here in light of the individual's reaction to the group is the question: do individuals choose reference groups, and must certain reference group membership be acknowledged regardless of the individual's desire to claim this group as a reference group. It is clear that individuals can and do adopt new reference groups throughout their lifetime. It is also clear that individuals often wish to denounce certain reference groups or referent others with whom they ordinarily would be associated, such as a racial or ethnic group. Certain ethnic and racial groups, for example, carry with them a negative social identification. Such is true in our society with various minority groups. Is it possible for members to escape their affiliations with these groups? In these cases "membership" is established at birth. What is the nature of his adaptation to a reference group to which he does not want to belong? These are questions that will be taken up more fully in a discussion of the destructive reference group affiliations that a member acquires.

Although a reference group may be a negative source of identification, as is suggested above, reference groups do serve as positive sources of identification and offer a number of benefits to members. Membership in reference groups does not always mean that one has a negative source of identification, that his belonging to a group is both undesirable and carries a negative connotation in the society at large. Quite frequently individuals choose referent others to enhance their self-concepts. Membership in certain occupational groups, for example, often carry prestige and status that is felt by the individual in terms of increased self-esteem and greater feelings of self-worth.

In addition to providing an individual with a positive source of identification, the reference group enables one to formulate a distinct identity. Belonging to a reference group tends to locate the individual with respect to the larger society, which is often made up of an array of possible identities. He gains a specific identity by being a member; that is, for example, he is a Jew, or a longshoreman, or a black man. This identity he shares with others in a group of Jews, longshoremen, or black men, respectively. In his search for who he is not, who he is, and how he should behave, he continually views himself with respect to his membership in this group. He has a basis of identity through his membership in the group. Essentially his self-image is established and reaffirmed from day to day in interaction with others of the same and different reference groups.[10] Individuals who lack identification with a specific reference group, who are changing their referent others, or who experience conflict between various reference groups to which they belong, feel the nebulous sense of a lack of a specific identity associated with the absence of a clearly defined and unconflicted reference group membership. These persons sometimes ramble aimlessly and anxiously through relationships looking for themselves, in essence, for a location or identity in the society at large. Secondary to a lack of reference group ties is also the problem of role diffusion—of not knowing what to be (essentially because one does not know who he is and what values are most important). (See Erik H. Erikson's *Childhood and Society*.[3])

Reference groups also meet individuals' need for homonymy. A sense of belonging, of continuity and sameness with the outside world associated with knowing one is like others, yet a sense of being autonomous or separate and self-directing is described by many social psychologists, among whom is Daniel Adelson,[1] as necessary in the makeup of any normal individual. Persons who lack either a sense of homonymy (of being like others) or a sense of autonomy (of being unique and self-directed) are sometimes those individuals who suffer moderate to severe emotional disturbance. It is not clear whether emotional disturbance is a result or a cause of a lack of reference group ties, for individuals who are deeply disturbed are also less likely to view themselves as members of a reference group and often withdraw from interaction with groups in the society at large. Still the correlation is impressive and warrants further investigation.

What does seem clear is that individuals who do claim reference groups also benefit by having their needs for homonymy met, needs essential to their self-concept and feelings of security. Although some persons misuse this membership, for example, become overly dependent on their reference group as a source of identity to the point of complete loss of a unique identity, the value of reference group membership to individuals is unquestionable.

It has been noted that individuals may belong to several reference groups throughout their lifetime and that a process of choosing and changing reference groups and referent others goes on. Why and how one changes and chooses reference groups is an interesting phenomena and one worth exploring further. Shibutani[10] and others note that individuals have many reference groups but that their ties to these groups vary. When one acquires a new reference group, he establishes a new audience and standard of conduct against which he measures himself. One conclusion then is that former standards of conduct may be perceived as undesirable for him or inadequate in meeting his personal needs; therefore the individual chooses new reference groups or referent others. This process may occur with adolescents who join teenage cliques despite former identification with their families and the sometimes contradictory values that are espoused by each of these groups.

Whenever an individual's status changes, for example, from a blue collar worker to a white collar worker, he acquires a new reference group. He learns new roles and his concept of himself becomes modified to incorporate new referent others. A change of status, such as with a job promotion, is often the result of the individual's own desire to increase his status and prestige.

What seems to be common to individuals' changing and choosing reference groups are (1) some desire on the part of the individual to satisfy unmet needs, for example, for greater status or for standards of conduct fitting his personal growth and development needs and (2) a necessary replacement of former significant others with new significant others, or simply the acquisition of significant others. (This is the case of the infant whose immediate reference group, and essentially one of his first, is his family—more particularly his parents.) New significant others usually represent the point of view that the individual accepts as his own. The displacement of a former reference group by a new one indicates that the individual is redefining himself and taking on new perspectives. The adoption of a new perspective often makes it possible for individuals to reexamine and redefine the self. Therefore it would seem that individuals who do take on new reference groups, a process that is partially unconsciously motivated, want an opportunity to redefine themselves. It would also seem, however, that many individuals inherit reference group member-ships, for example, at birth, that may not be desirable. Being a member of a minority group may not be desirable at some point in one's life. Opportunities to redefine oneself in these latter cases may be unavailable to members. Still they may attempt to displace these reference groups. Members may change their names from Cohen to Hill or may attempt to "pass" as white.

The potential effects of reference group membership on an individual's overall concept of self and his adjustment seem to be quite dramatic. Certain reference groups, as was pointed out, can either enhance or lower his self-esteem.

Many psychotherapists contend that the essence of therapy is in fact the replace-ment of a low self-esteem and poor self-concept with a more favorable one. This, they claim, happens when individuals enter therapy and replace former significant others with new significant others, those who share values related to health and who can sustain more cordial interpersonal relations with the client.

Changes such as this were also seen to be the result of some growth and self-ac-tualization groups experience. Sherwood,[9] myself,[7] and others have noted changes in self-identity occurring as a result of membership in sensitivity groups. I found an increase in self-esteem in particular after members had sustained contact with each other in a sensitivity group. Members valued one another and the group as a whole more than at the outset of the group. One proposition in many of these studies is that the individual's self-identity and self-evaluation is dependent on his subjectively held version of peers' ratings of him. Sherwood indicated that changes which did oc-cur were also dependent on the differential importance of various peers for individu-als, the extent to which peer perceptions were communicated, and the individual's degree of involvement in the group.

In addition to these studies there is a great deal of literature that suggests one's membership in various reference groups does affect one's preferences and attitudes toward the self. The well-known study by Clark and Clark[2] with respect to the racial identification of black children is certainly a classic on this subject and indicates how identification with one's reference group may result in dislike for oneself and preference for objects associated with a different reference group.

Although the scope and nature of various forms of reference group memberships have not been explored fully enough to type or categorize them, the following is an attempt at some system of classification. It is believed that reference groups—familial, occupational, ethnic—may not differ radically from one another (except perhaps to the extent that these groups are inherited or acquired reference groups); they probably serve common purposes for the individual and may be responded to in the same ways. A classification, however, that does seem to be helpful and that does shed light on the variations which may occur with reference groups is one that looks to the nature of the membership, that is, to whether it is a constructive or destructive membership for the individual in terms of his identity formation, role adjustment, and self-concept.

Destructive affiliations

Reference group affiliations that (1) divide the self, as opposed to enhancing self-integration, (2) instill a low self-esteem, or (3) cause an imbalance in the satisfaction of needs for homonymy and autonomy may be referred to as those that lead to destructive reference group membership. Examples of such affiliation may involve membership with a group whose own values are conflicting, affiliation with one or more groups whose values conflict,[8] affiliation with a group that is devalued by the society at large, and excessive affiliation with a group so that one's unique identity is overshadowed. In each of these cases the nature of the reference group affiliation, as well as the identity the group carries with it, operates to make the membership destructive to the individual.

Reference group affiliations that prohibit a sufficient balance of homonymy and autonomy may be observable in several different instances. Such affiliation either is not strong enough to give individuals a sense of belonging in the society at large, or else is too strong and denies the individual any uniqueness he may have of his own. In our society many individuals strive for an identity through group affiliation, but in doing so they "lose themselves." Typical examples of this may be seen with various cults or cliques that develop among youth but also among adults, for example, the middle class suburban housewife groups. It is not unusual to observe that members of these reference groups deny any unique identification they might have, above and beyond that which fits the standards of the group. Members may dress alike, talk alike, do the same things, and live by the same standards and values. Interestingly enough it is such groups that are now flocking to self-actualization groups in numbers.[10] It would seem that they are either trying to reverse the effects of their current membership in their reference groups, or they have simply substituted one dependency for another and have found a new "cult."

Reference groups that bestow a certain negative self-concept on their members are also potentially destructive to the individual. These are groups that decrease individuals' self-esteem, chiefly because as members of these groups, individuals take on the negative connotation of the group held by members of the society at large. More specifically, certain racial, ethnic, occupational, and religious groups have acquired a negative image in our society. Being a member of these groups elicits certain prejudices from others. The plight of our minorities is well noted in the litera-ture in texts like Grier and Cobbs' *Black Rage*[4] and in such novels as Griffin's *Black Like Me*.[5] Reference groups, then, that instill in their members a negative self-image most frequently cause the individual lowered self-esteem. Individuals may respond by denying their affiliation with their referent others, by fighting the present status of the group, that is, by trying to enhance the prestige of the group, or by accepting the negative identity, in despair, as that of their own. Nonetheless, individuals suffer from the fact that as members of the group they inherit an array of prejudices and a negative self-image that is both difficult to incorporate in one's own image of self and difficult to escape.

A third and final type of destructive reference group affiliation is that which di-vides the self. As mentioned earlier, this type of affiliation may be the result of identi-fication with a group that has conflicting values of its own or identification with two or more groups that have conflicting values and standards. Noncomplimentary inter-action of two or more reference groups is common in our society with the variety of roles and identifications from which to choose.[10] Affiliations in groups whose values or expectations are conflicting with one another often lead to part-time identifica-tions. For example, individuals who come from a blue collar background and who have recently broken into a white collar profession may associate only with middle and upper-middle class members of their profession while at work, but on weekends they may prefer to dress, act, and associate with common laborers. In our society, roles of mother and wife conflict with those of an occupation or profession. Women may identify with both groups of referent others—mothers and wives, as well as per-sons of a certain profession. The values and expectations of one group are known to differ and sometimes conflict with those of the other group. Again, to mediate these differences the individual may maintain parttime identifications with both groups. Affiliation of this kind rarely provides individuals an opportunity to integrate their various self-images. As a whole it tends to perpetuate a lack of integration and differ-ential responses to oneself, depending on what role one is occupying at the time.

The consequences of destructive membership may be seen in individuals' over-all role adjustment, identity formation, and self-esteem. Individuals who maintain destructive reference group affiliations often have a vague or contradictory sense of who they are and what they should do.[6] They frequently choose and respond to dif-ferent roles, whether these roles are occupational or familial, with a lack of assur-ance about self. They might come to the attention of health professionals and others as the misguided, misplaced, and misjudged role occupants in our society. They of-ten have a low self-esteem, lack awareness of their unique individual attributes, and hold conflicting beliefs about what they should do or how they should act. Although it is probable that many of these individuals do come in contact with professional mental health services, it is also likely that many float in and around health and wel-fare agencies never explicitly asking for help and often being aided in inappropriate ways.

The role of the nurse in aiding individuals who have maintained destructive ref-erence group affiliations borders on that of a therapeutic agent who possesses various skills related to therapy and counseling. Nurses are best equipped to help these individuals if (1) they have an established and integrated identity through group membership, (2) they have had a strong theoretical and clinical background in growth and development (especially identity formation), and (3) they have had some preparation in counseling persons with problems of low self-esteem and identity conflict. As therapeutic agents with these individuals they may employ several methods to help individuals with reference to conflicts they may have. They may help them determine which set of values is most personally desirable or which expectations fit the individuals' unique capacities. They may help them acquire an altered self-concept that would elevate their self-esteem. They may, for example, point out the person's good points and support the individual's attempts to counter the image he has acquired. The nurse, then, can serve as a therapeutic agent with those who have maintained or acquired destructive reference group memberships. Many other reference group memberships seem to necessitate little or no intervention on the part of a nurse or other health professional. These affiliations may be referred to as constructive reference group memberships.

Constructive affiliations

Constructive reference group memberships are those that (1) integrate various perceptions of the self,[6] (2) afford a balance in autonomy and homonymy, and (3) lead to increased or high self-esteen. Reference groups that foster positive growth in members have (1) commonly shared goals, where group *and individual* goals are encouraged, (2) an accepting, collaborative atmosphere that supports change, (3) a philosophy that encourages the individual to take responsibility for his own growth even though he identifies with the group, (4) standards that support each member, serving as a resource to help others in the group, and (5) communication that allows for establishment of common meanings and feelings of solidarity. Constructive membership may result from identification with a group holding unconflicting expectations complimentary to the individual's own self-perception, from the fact that the identification does not overshadow one's personal uniqueness and still gives the individual a sense of belonging, or from identification with a group that bestows a positive self-image to the individual.

Reference group memberships that increase members' self-esteem are examples of the latter type of affiliation. An individual who is a member of a certain reference group may inherit a number of desirable self-referents, for example, courage, beauty, intelligence, humaneness. These are qualities of the group that are attributed to its members as well. These qualities may be associated with certain occupational groups for example. Being a member of a group that itself elicits high regard guarantees the individual a higher self-regard. Also, groups formed to achieve some approved or admired goal but which have not met this goal are still sources of high regard.

Group membership that allows members to meet both their needs for autonomy and for homonymy are constructive memberships. Individuals neither depend on the group for their entire self-definition nor do groups demand this of them. Still the group may assign them a special identity in the society at large. Persons who are self-actualized who feel a certain unity with their surroundings and yet a separateness with respect to their own individuality have usually developed constructive reference group affiliations. In some instances these persons are regarded as the mature, self-potentialized members of the society.

Lastly, reference group memberships that act to integrate the individual's sense of self with various expectations and values of the group may be referred to as constructive affiliations. If the individual belongs to more than one group, the standards of these groups are usually complimentary and also reflect the individual's own expectations of self. Consequently members experience increased feelings of self-assurance: they know who they are and where they are going and suffer few self-doubts.[6] Essentially they make up the segment of the community that is goal directed, self-assured, and self-directive. Quite frequently then, they are the "model" citizens and leaders of the community.

The consequences of constructive reference group membership have already been alluded too. These consequences have to do with an individual's self-concept, identity formation, and role adjustment. Individuals who maintain constructive reference group memberships have a clear and unconflicted sense of who they are and what they should do. They choose and respond to different roles with deliberation and self-assurance. Expectations of the self are usually matched by those of the reference group. Essentially they are the role occupants who demonstrate a sense of fitness and a positive level of self-esteem. It is rare that these individuals will need professional counseling or therapy, even in light of normal life crises. What then should be the role of the health professional with respect to constructive reference group affiliations?

If one assumes that constructive group affiliations can be acquired and are sometimes created from more adverse situations, then one can foresee a role for a therapeutic agent such as the nurse or nurse-counselor. Constructive group affiliations that provide for both the individual's needs for autonomy and homonymy depend in part on the individual's own response to his various reference groups. The nurse can encourage him to strive for a unique identity if he is dependent on his reference group for identification. Specifically nurses can help the individual identify those attributes of his that set him apart from others. If the individual is detached from any reference group whatsoever, the nurse can help him explore various groups suited to him and to his interests, needs, and concerns.

In addition, nurses can encourage memberships in groups that are not conflicting with respect to their values and standards. In part this is a task of helping the individual determine which set of values are most important to him. If individuals do not seem to be able to break ties with these groups, despite the fact that their standards are conflictual, the nurse is obliged to help the individual recognize that his own frustrations lie within a conflict in expectations or values of these groups, and that consequences are likely to result in such things as part-time identification with these groups. Knowledge or awareness of this type is at least supportive of the individual who is experiencing feelings of being pulled in two different directions without knowing what is happening to him.

Lastly the nurse is in a position to recommend groups or clubs to individuals that are likely to enhance their self-esteem. Goal-oriented groups, those which have an admired objective (for example, hospital volunteer groups) can afford members increased self-esteem.

Whether in informal counseling sessions or in more structured formal therapeutic relationships, the nurse has a role in both mediating the consequences of destructive reference group memberships and in enhancing the acquisition of more constructive reference group memberships. Unlike other therapeutic and group therapy groups, the reference group has not been appreciated nor recognized for its effects on members. Still, as was pointed out here, these memberships have a number of consequences with respect to individuals' identity formation, role adjustment, and self-concept. Reference groups are pervasive throughout one's lifetime. Indirectly or directly, nurses as therapeutic agents will deal with the fact that their clients or patients identify with various reference groups or referent others. These identifications may be more or less constructive. The nurse must be able to identify certain helpful and more destructive elements of these identifications, as well as be prepared to intervene in a meaningful way, either to enhance constructive affiliations or to modify the effects of destructive reference group memberships.

REFERENCES

1. Adelson, D.: Lectures from psychology 200, University of California Medical Center, San Francisco, 1967.
2. Clark, K. B., and Clark, M. P.: Racial identification and preference in Negro children. In Newcomb, T., and Hurtley, E., editors: Readings in social psychology, New York, 1947, Henry Holt & Co., pp. 169-178.
3. Erikson, E. H.: Childhood and society, New York, 1950, W. W. Norton & Co.
4. Grier, W. H., and Cobbs, P. M.: Black rage, London, 1969, Jonathan Cape Ltd.
5. Griffin, J. H.: Black like me, Boston, 1961, Houghton Mifflin Co.
6. Lecky, P.: Self-consistency: a theory of personality (edited and interpreted by F. C. Thorne), Hamden, Conn., 1961, The Shoe String Press.
7. Marram, G.: What is happening to nurses? Int. Nurs. Rev. **16:**320-328, 1969.
8. Miller, D., and Swanson, G.: Inner conflict and defense, New York, 1960, Holt, Rinehart & Winston.
9. Sherwood, J. J.: Self-identity and referent others, Sociometry **28:**66-81, 1965.
10. Shibutani, T.: Society and personality—an interactionist approach to social psychology, Englewood Cliffs, N.J., 1961, Prentice-Hall.

SUGGESTED READINGS
Introduction
Asch, S.: Opinions and social pressure. In Rosenbaum, M., and Berger, M., editors: Group psychotherapy and group function, ed. 2, New York, 1975, Basic Books, Inc., Publishers.
Bugental, J. F. T., and Zelen, S. L.: Investigations into the self concept, J. Pers. **18:**438-498, 1950.
Goffman, E.: The presentation of self in everyday life, Garden City, N.Y., 1959, Doubleday & Co.
Papanek, H.: Therapeutic and antitherapeutic factors in group relations, Am. J. Psychother. **23:** 396-404, 1969.
Rosenberg, M.: Society and the adolescent self-image, Princeton, N.J., 1965, Princeton University Press.
Sanford, N.: Self and society, New York, 1966, Atherton Press.

Sherif, M.: The self and reference groups, Ann. N.Y. Acad. Sci. **96:**681-894, 1962.
Wiley, R. C.: The self concept: a critical survey of pertinent research, Lincoln, Nebr., 1961, University of Nebraska Press.

Destructive affiliations

Allport, G. W.: The nature of prejudice, Cambridge, Mass., 1954, Addison-Wesley Publishing Co.
Bosselman, B. C.: Self-destruction: a study of suicidal impulses, Springfield, Ill., 1958, Charles C Thomas, Publisher.
Cohen, A. K.: Delinquent boys: the culture of the gang, Glencoe, Ill., 1955, The Free Press, pp. 151-299.

Constructive affiliations

Crutchfield, R. A.: Independent thought in a conformist world. In Farber, S., and Wilson, R. H., editors: Conflict and creativity, New York, 1963, McGraw-Hill Book Co.
Dunkas, N., and Nikelly, A.: Group psychotherapy with Greek immigrants, Int. J. Group Psychother. **25:**402-409, 1975.
Grold, J.: The value of a youth group to hospitalized adolescents. In Berkovitz, I., editor: Adolescents grow in groups, New York, 1975, Brunner/Mazel.
McDonald, T.: Group psychotherapy with native American women, Int. J. Group Psychother. **25:**410-420, 1975.

MATCHING EXERCISE FOR PART ONE

As a review of Part One, try matching *individual(s)* with their *needs* and the appropriate *group* experience. There may be more than one correct response in each case. When matching these examples be aware of the process or rationale you use in reaching a decision.

Individuals

I. A 30-year-old lawyer concerned with not being authentic, his "true self"

II. A 45-year-old woman who had corrective surgery of the bowel, necessitating a colostomy

III. A 55-year-old woman who has gone from doctor to doctor seeking a diet to help her lose 60 pounds and who is always discouraged because doctors reprimand her

IV. A 12-year-old girl whose emotional problems relate to the fact that her mother is depressed and seeks her support

V. A 28-year-old housewife who has just acknowledged she has a drinking problem but does not know where to turn for help

VI. Seventh-grade junior high school group of students exploring issues about sex

VII. A 57-year-old chronic schizophrenic, paranoid-type female patient hospitalized over 12 years in the back ward of a state hospital

VIII. A 40-year-old manager of a firm whose staff is concerned that they have no say in making decisions that affect them

IX. A 65-year-old man who has just been admitted to a nursing home and suffers transient depression due to the loss of his wife a year ago

X. A couple with marriage problems, one spouse being a discharged mental patient

XI. A 45-year-old energetic construction worker with cardiac problems who was rehospitalized because he does not follow his doctor's regimen of rest and moderation.

XII. A 27-year-old woman who was just admitted to a county hospital receiving ward in an acute catatonic stupor

Needs

a. To identify with others in a group in order to curb undesirable impulses

b. To develop increased sensitivity to others and enhance one's interpersonal competence

c. To respond to others in new ways in order to realize capacities and limitations that have been hidden by everyday roles and masquerades

d. To adjust to the fact that one's bodily functions have been interrupted but that there are ways to compensate

e. To have sustained contact with one other mental health professional

f. To realize one's realistic capacities to function through associations with others who face the same handicap

g. To examine the array of behavioral opportunities possible and the consequences of each

h. To learn alternative ways of relating to one other significant other that are not detrimental to either party

i. To acquire former social skills abandoned because of sustained isolation

j. To meet with others who have suffered losses in order to share with one another feelings of frustration and loneliness

k. To seek relief from one's own stress through the treatment of himself and others close to him

Groups

1. Growth and self-actualization groups (e.g., encounter, sensitivity, marathon, and group dynamics groups)

2. Self-help groups (e.g., AA, Synanon, TOPS, and laryngectomy clubs)

3. Therapeutic groups (e.g., with the hospitalized, aged, school children, and in the community at large)

4. Group therapy or psychotherapy groups (e.g., with psychiatric inpatients, outpatients, families, and couples or milieu therapy)

5. Reference groups (e.g., constructive affiliations)

6. No group experience is appropriate at this time

ANSWERS

It may be helpful to refer back to various sections of Part One to determine how soundly based your decisions are. The following is one list of possible matches of individuals, needs, and appropriate group experiences.

I, c, 1	VII, i, 4
II, d, 2	VIII, b, 1
III, a, 2	IX, j, 3
IV, k, 4	X, h, 4
V, a, 2	XI, f, 3
VI, g, 3	XII, e, 6

PART TWO

Theoretical orientations behind the study and practice of group work

Nurses, as they become involved in group work, will be guided not only by their own interests but also by their particular skills and knowledges. In some group work they will be expected to have rather specific skills and knowledges related to psychotherapy and psychopathology. Essential to their practicing group work of any kind is a basic understanding of themselves and of how they operate in a group situation, as well as a theoretical framework that will guide their interpretations about the group and their interventions. The theoretical framework on which they base their interpretations and interventions may draw from any number of psychiatric, psychological, and social psychological thoughts and may include psychoanalytic, interpersonal, communication, group dynamics, existential, Gestalt, and behavioral modification theories. Although nurses may favor one theory over the others, they may find that an eclectic orientation is more helpful and in some cases more appropriate, especially if they wish to operate in a variety of groups. Nurses must know what benefits can be expected from group experience and how to intervene in a meaningful therapeutic manner to ensure that these benefits are operant for the individuals in their group at various stages of group development. In addition there are special knowledges nurses may need in conducting a group. These include knowledge and skill in coleading and knowledge of particular techniques that can be employed in group work, as well as a knowledge of how roles evolve and function in a group setting.

Part Two of this text focuses on theoretical frameworks that guide our study and practice in group work. The total number of theoretical models are not exhausted in this discussion. Rather, I have chosen key theories that may be explored singularly and in further depth if the nurse chooses to adapt one framework. If not, certain concepts and principles from each framework can be combined to provide the leader with a practical eclectic approach modifiable by the specific patient population one is working with.

CHAPTER 6

An overview

Introduction

The study and practice of group work can draw upon a wide range of theoretical frameworks and schools of thought. This is to be expected, since the practice of group work focuses on individuals in group settings, as well as on the properties of a group per se. In this sense it is a fertile ground for traditional and modern psychological and psychotherapeutic thought, ranging from psychoanalytic to existential perspectives and including theories of group dynamics, communication, and behavioral modification.

The purpose of this chapter is to explore the scope of the various theoretical schools of thought that are frequently applied in the study and practice of group work in a variety of group settings. The appropriateness of any one theory with respect to the focus and goals of the group may vary, but at least one of the theories discussed here will be relevant to any group, whether it be medical-surgical patients anticipating surgery, unwed mothers coping with problems of social isolation, or patients in a community mental health center. Since some theories are only indirectly applicable, in-depth discussion would lead away from the primary focus on groups per se and from the application of a theory. The reader is encouraged, however, to expand his knowledge of the theories discussed here if more than a broad analytical basis for group work is desired.

To this point the assumption has been made, but not put to a test, that a theory for the practice and study of group work is both relevant and important.

Before discussing selected theories, it is helpful to consider arguments for and against a theoretical basis for group work itself. By theoretical basis is meant a compilation of logically interlinked concepts and principles that help to explain or predict certain phenomena. One theory, for example, may explain why a member reacts as he does or what will happen at different stages of the group.

It is possible that explanations applied to group practice are not necessary and hamper the leader's ability to facilitate the group's development. In certain respects, knowledge of group theory on the part of the leader is not necessary for members to reap benefits from their participation. Some benefits that come from participating seem to occur without the leader's knowledge and utilization of a particular theory to guide his interventions. A theory is often regarded by novices as a barrier to their understanding and to their ability to be effective. Beginning nurse practitioners have complained to me that if they concentrate on projecting a theory to the group, they miss what seems to be the essence of its interaction. In part this problem relates to the fact that they lack experience in leadership as well as a complete understanding of the particular theory. But also this problem relates to the fact that theories can be inadequate in describing group phenomena.

If theories do not capture the essence of group interaction or fail to consider how multiple forces interact, they are deemed irrelevant to group work. In short, theories can oversimplify what is actually going on. Because they can also act as a barrier to the leader's perception of the "whole," they are sometimes accused of being useless and of hampering the leader's ability to be effective.

On the other hand, it can also be argued that a theory is relevant and essential and should therefore be employed by all group practitioners. The ability to explain and predict phenomena can aid leaders in reaching their goals more efficiently and effectively. In addition group leaders must have some basis of determining what events are conducive to their meeting their goals. Once involved with this problem, they are faced with the need to clarify and predict certain phenomena, therefore the need for a theory.

Arguments which imply that all group practitioners should operate within some theoretical framework are those concerned with the problems of promoting the practice of group work and its establishment as a professional modality. A theory about group development that also lends itself to implementation may be more easily communicated to others than specific esoteric ideas that have no logical framework. Practices supported by these theories are also more likely to be sustained than those that are not. In addition the mark of a profession is in part the extent to which it possesses a body of knowledge related to the expertise of its members. This is not simply any body of knowledge, but one that is empirically sound and logically based. Theories are the essential ingredients of this body of knowledge.

It is erroneous to conclude that a theory is irrelevant or unimportant to group research. Those who claim they are not operating within some theoretical framework are most likely mistaken; rather the underlying bases for their interventions may not be apparent. Even the inexperienced layman who somehow becomes involved in group work is guided by some systematic process by which he determines when and how to intervene as a leader. Most leaders cannot ignore for long such questions as: What makes persons act the way they do in the group? Does the group have a life of its own—independent of what individuals contribute? Once they entertain answers to these questions, they are formulating a theory about groups and group practice.

The development of a theoretical basis has, however, had its problems. To a large extent the development of theories to fit group work has been haphazard, resembling the process of developing a theory to fit any applied discipline. Part of the problem lies with our inability to develop an overriding theoretical framework that can be implemented in studying many groups. This dilemma confronts the nursing profession to some extent. Several attempts to develop such a theoretical framework, which can be implemented in nursing as well as group work, are in danger of being so general that they lose all meaning for the practitioner or omit important features of the practitioner's role.

Theories regarding group work not only have faced the problem of being either too specific or too general but also are constantly subjected to certain trends and fads that occur in their "parent" disciplines—the behavioral sciences. Group theories have undergone at least two major shifts in focus within the last three decades. Essentially theories have shifted from an emphasis on the individual for the purpose of personality reconstruction (largely in the 1950s) to a focus on individual self-actualization (largely in the 1960s to the present) and then to a focus on the group as a center for solving specific problems, for example, racial tension (largely in the late 1960s and early 1970s and into the future).

The development of group theories is not exclusively the domain of psychology or any other single science. Theorists and practitioners from many disciplines, including nursing, business, sociology, social work, communication, and urban development are contributing, invited or not, to the array of theories about group work. This fact makes the problem of establishing a predominant theory even more out of reach.

Having briefly considered the problems of the development of a theoretical framework for group work and discussed the arguments for and against a theoretical basis for its study and practice, we now move to an examination of several theories appropriate for different types of groups. The reader will note that in some instances the division between one framework and another is only arbitrary. In fact one framework may be derived from another; but for the purposes of this discussion, differences between these frameworks will be highlighted, respecting the framework of their origin.

Psychoanalytic framework

It is not surprising that various established theories of psychology and individual behavior have an impact on theories germane to group work. Perhaps the most obvious reason for this influence is that therapeutic problems of individuals in the group seem so closely parallel to those of persons involved in individual therapy of various types.

Although Freud and classic freudian psychologists are best known for contributions in the area of individual psychology, Freud and his followers made "innovative" and provocative claims in reference to group psychology and practice. Among current practitioners and theorists who are committed to a psychoanalytic framework applied to group practice are Slavson,[18] Wolfe and Schwartz,[22] Ezriel,[9] and other Tavistock Clinic (London) theorists. These practitioners and theorists adhere to one or more of the traditional psychoanalytic principles: (1) the existence of unconscious motives, (2) the symbolic reenactment of the past in present relationships with others, (3) the existence of basic love-hate instincts, and (4) a topographical description of the mind consisting of three distinct divisions—the id, the ego, and the superego. We will discuss these principles in sequence and relate them to the study and practice of group work.

Existence of unconscious motives

The psychoanalytic premise that an unconscious basis for an individual's behavior actually exists is easily transcribed to the group setting. For example, if an unconscious basis for one individual's behavior exists, then the behavior of individuals in a group as a whole is to some extent motivated or modified by unconscious processes, that is, needs, desires, or fears. The unconscious, which Freud called Pandora's box, includes elements barred from access to consciousness. What many theorists today refer to as unconscious elements of behavior are actually more accurately referred to as those elements that are temporarily latent, or, what Freud claimed, located in the preconscious. When we discuss unconscious manifestations of members' behavior in a group, we are actually including those elements Freud would have referred to as preconscious, meaning that which, given the individual's attention, can be brought to consciousness with little effort.

Practitioners and theorists who recognize the unconscious manifestations of an individual's behavior within the group loosely refer to his actual behavior as the manifest content and to his underlying motives or covert forces as the latent content.

Ezriel,[9] Whitaker and Liebermann,[21] and others of the Tavistock Clinic developed extensive theories on group interaction based on the principles of latent content. They added a new dimension and refined the concept of unconscious motivation for an individual's behavior in a group setting. Essentially they proposed the existence of a "group unconscious"; that is, they suggested that not only are unconscious motives relevant to a single individual's behavior within the group but also that what governs group process and movement may be the unconscious fears and desires of the group as a collective body of individuals. Underlying this idea of a group unconscious is the premise that a group has a "mind" of its own. This premise is embedded in other theories about groups and will be discussed later in this chapter.

Whitaker and Liebermann[21] are most renowned for their elucidation of what they call nuclear conflicts and group focal conflicts. These conflicts describe the unconscious fears and desires of individuals, as well as those of the group as a whole.

Nuclear conflicts are those peculiar to the individual and are what each individual brings to the group from his earlier life experiences. They consist of (1) a disturbing motive or wish; (2) a reactive motive or corresponding fear; and (3) a solution that the individual employs to maximize fulfillment of his wish yet protect himself from what he fears. The solution he employs is usually habitual and one that the individual will seek to maintain in the group. An example of a nuclear conflict manifested in the group could be an individual's desire to have a unique relationship with the group leader, yet possess a corresponding fear of criticism and condemnation by other members. A solution that the individual may employ to maximize fulfillment of his wish, yet protect himself from what he fears, would be to remain after the group encounters to have "private" conversations with the leader about how the group is going. His nuclear conflict and the solutions he employs are beyond his awareness.

When individual and total group concerns become interdependent, a group focal conflict may arise. Such a conflict is composed of shared desires or fears and agreed on solutions. Whitaker and Liebermann[21] claimed that the initial focal conflicts are generally a result of members' expectations of the group, its structure and composition. Certain disturbing motives that can characterize beginning group sessions are wishes (1) to reveal one's problems in the group; (2) to please the leader; (3) to have a special relationship with the leader; and (4) to form intimate relationships with others in the group. Early reactive motives or shared fears are likely to include fears of criticism or ridicule from the other members, fears of harm through contact with other people who have problems, fears of hurting other members, fears of punishment or retaliation from the leader or other members, and fears of intolerable guilt or anxiety. Group solutions to these conflicts may take the form of (1) coping with the conflict by avoiding recognition that the feelings belong to oneself, for example, members denying that they want a special relationship with the leader, (2) recognizing their desires but rationalizing them as a group, for example, claiming that it is normal for members to want the leader to like them, (3) safely expressing their wish so that the feared consequences will not occur, for example, getting everyone to reveal their problems in the group, (4) or getting the leader to provide a solution, for example, asking the leader to control things or to make a ruling against retaliation by other members. Group focal conflicts, like nuclear conflicts, are beyond the awareness of the group.

The role of the leader in a group where focal conflicts arise is basically to facilitate members' recognition of their desires and fears, as well as of the particular solutions that the group employs to cope with its conflicts. Whitaker and Liebermann claim that a knowledge of these unconscious forces enables the leader to (1) examine group process and individual involvement from an analytical point of view, (2) view individual and total group concerns as interdependent, and (3) choose interventions that increase members' awareness of their conflicts and of more successful solutions to these conflicts, thus indirectly aiding the individual to alter his particular nuclear conflict.

In Chapter 10, case study 3, the reader will find a detailed discussion of the concept of focal conflict as it applies to leader assessment and intervention in a group.

Symbolic reenactment of the past in present relationships

Perhaps the most popular theorist today in respect to symbolic reenactment of the past in present relationships with others, yet also writing with groups in mind, is Eric Berne. Berne has contributed several texts that outline his approach to groups and psychoanalysis. Among these are *A Layman's Guide to Psychiatry and Psychoanalysis*,[4] *Transactional Analysis in Psychotherapy*,[5] and *Principles of Group Treatment*.[3] Berne's theory is essentially designed to apply to group therapy but also is used for group work with a variety of persons, ranging from adolescents and more well-adjusted individuals to psychotics, psychopaths, and psychosomatic patients. Berne directs his theory specifically to the nature of members' behavior as it relates to symbolic reenactment of the past in present relationships.

Essentially Berne's approach to analyzing members' participation involves his schema of adult, child, and parent roles. Berne[5] suggests that within each group situation, members symbolically reenact former problems by relating to others certain complimentary roles. For example, the interaction between members 1 and 2 may be that which is typical between a child and his parent. Member 1 may respond to member 2 as if 2 were his parent; he may, for example, interpret 2's remarks as protective or censoring. Usually there is something about 1's behavior that elicits 2's tendency toward responding as a parent. Member 1 may look fragile or may rebel in the group and thereby elicit feelings and behavior from 2 that are typical parent-like responses. The fact that the members' interaction is heavily ladened with emotions may give the leader a clue that members are reenacting what occurred in former relationships.

Berne maintains that childhood ego states exist as relics in the adult and that under certain circumstances they can be revived. Persons can be observed to shift from one state of mind and one behavior to another. Berne explains that an individual can engage in reality testing and rational thinking, aspects of what Freud[10] described as secondary process, or in autistic thinking and archaic fears and expectations, what Freud referred to as primary process. The former, Berne concludes, has the quality of the usual mode of functioning for responsible adults, whereas the latter resembles the behavior of young children. Berne conceptualizes the former as adult and the latter as child manifestations of the individual in the group.

A state that fits neither of these two categories but that is reminiscent of the way an individual's parents had seemed to him is what Berne refers to as the parent ego state. Persons are capable, then, of imitating their father's or mother's behavior in the group through their interaction with the other members. To summarize, Berne asserts that members can reenact the past in their present relationships with group members. They may shift from child, parent, or adult, depending on stimuli they receive in their interaction. Member 1 may elicit a response from member 2; this response becomes a stimulus for member 1 or other members. Responses from member 1 or other members become new stimuli for member 2.

Berne claims that once the leader can sufficiently type the responses of members interacting together as parent, child, or adult, then the rest of the interaction between members is highly predictable. Essentially it will follow the initial pattern established until the stimuli that members receive are strikingly different from those received thus far, or until the roles they have been portraying are no longer appropriate. Berne believes the leader can develop a keen awareness of the problems of members and of the nature of the group interaction by employing these transactional principles. Once the leader has an understanding of the individuals in respect to the roles they have assumed and of the nature of the interaction in the group, he has the ability to alter what is occurring and to assist individuals in choosing more desirable roles in their interaction with others. The leader has the option then of (1) stopping the pattern of interaction established, (2) pointing out to members how they are participating—as the child, parent, or adult, (3) aiding members in seeing how their behavior is in part a result of their perceptions of others in the group and of significant interaction with others in the past, and (4) assisting them in evaluating the desirability of their roles and the nature of group interaction, in hopes that they will test other roles and means of interacting with each other which are more desirable to individual members and the group as a whole.

Existence of basic love-hate instincts

Slavson,[18] as well as other group analysts, adheres to the principle of the existence of basic love-hate instincts that underlie an individual's interaction with others in a group setting. Initially related to Freud's concept of basic drives, the interpretation of love-hate instincts in group interaction takes on special meaning.

Freud directed his theory of basic drives to answering the problem of what motivates persons along constructive paths and what causes them to adapt destructive patterns of behavior. He was concerned with essentially two conditions—one can be categorized as the destructive instinct (thanatos) and the other as the constructive instinct (eros). These are also referred to as the love and death instincts. They are said to either work against each other or combine with each other. Freud defined libido as that energy which acts to neutralize an individual's destructive impulses which are thought to be simultaneously present in individuals. Slavson[18] and others claim that with some individuals, libido or life energy needs to be redistributed to the extent that feelings of hate, for example, do not predominate in their interaction with others and are neutralized by members' affection and appreciation of others and themselves. For example, if members behave in ways to elicit rejection from the group or display only hostile feelings toward the leader or other members, these individuals would seem to be dominated by their instincts for destruction. They would appear to be committed not only to self-destruction but also to destroying the group as a whole. Such destruction may take the form of blocking group movement per se or of severely criticizing the group to the extent that the group never achieves a sense of positive self-esteem or satisfaction. In this case it would be important for the leader and other members to mobilize these individuals' libidos in order to neutralize tendencies toward self- and group destruction.

Group dynamics theorists attribute to the group as a whole, instincts toward preservation and dissolution, rather than analyzing individuals' interaction in light of the existence of individual love-hate instincts. Group critics who stress the destructive potential of groups, and of sensitivity groups in particular, regard the group per se as deleterious to individuals. Ackerman[1] points out that groups are considered to encourage irrational behaviors and, in general, to be responsible for social ills, and therefore are destructive. This is a curious phenomenon, since the group is also a repository for civilized values and the source of control of destructive instincts. What Ackerman suggests is that if we regard a group as an individual having basic destructive impulses, we must also attribute to it basic healthy and constructive tendencies in regard to society's and individual members' well-being.

Existence of the id, ego, and superego

Psychoanalytic group theorists not only liken the group to an individual in respect to the existence of unconscious motives and basic constructive and destructive tendencies but also regard the group as possessing distinct functions that resemble the id, ego, and superego functions of the individual.

Originally Freud intended the description of id, ego, and superego to apply to a topography of the mind of the individual.[6] The id described the region of the mind that supposedly harbored repressed, primitive, and instinctive impulses concerned with the gratification of these impulses. Since it is not modified by reality, the id has often been equated with the term *unconscious*. Most of its contents are believed to never reach the level of conscious awareness. The ego is that region of the mind which brings the influence of the external world to bear on irrational impulses of the id and also functions to protect the self from too strong a superego. The superego is believed to have its roots in the prohibitions and ideals of the individual's parents, who imposed external threat of punishment, and later to operate regardless of parents' presence, as the adult has incorporated the parents' standards and values. The superego censors and rewards the individual in respect to his thoughts, feelings, and behavior.

Among those group theorists who attribute certain characteristics of the id, ego, and superego of the individual to the group is William Schutz.[17] Schutz expounds on the ego of a group in respect to the nature of its leadership. Schutz infers that ego functions of the individual in modifying irrational impulses and protecting the individual from too strong a superego are the functions of the group leader. Essentially the leader or members who take on leadership functions help the group adapt to reality and guide it toward rational goals. The leader should provide for members' needs; yet, if these needs are somehow incompatible with the here and now of the group (the external reality), the leader should help members modify their needs so that they are not detrimental to the total group function. For example, Schutz refers to the need for closeness and intimacy among members of the group. The leader's function in respect to this need is to allow for sufficient interpersonal closeness so that the group can feel the pleasures of friendship and affection, yet to modify the level of intimacy if the actions of members begin to distort the overall objectives. The leader modifies irrational wishes of the group by bringing to bear the outer reality. At the same time, the leader protects the group from too strong a superego, which would prevent members from meeting their needs completely. In this case members expressing the attitude that individuals should not get close to each other would take on the severe censoring role of the superego. When leadership functions are shared by various members and not assumed only by the official leader, members can be said to interact with each other in a manner typical to ego functioning.

Having highlighted some of the key concepts in psychoanalytic theory adapted to the study and practice of group work, we now turn to an examination of concepts which, although they can be said to be derivatives of psychoanalytic theory, are distinctly different and compose a framework referred to as interpersonal theory.

Interpersonal framework

The significance of interpersonal relationships in understanding and working with individuals within groups has preoccupied various group theorists since the advent of group work. Major importance has been attributed to the interpersonal theories of Harry Stack Sullivan and Frieda Fromm-Reichmann for at least a half century. The contributions that these theorists have made regarding a perspective on group work will be taken up as we discuss certain principles defined as interpersonal relationship-oriented. The reader will note as we present each theoretical framework that the boundaries we create between them are somewhat arbitrary and designed for the purpose of summarization and differentiation. The principles we will discuss include the following: (1) behavior, emotions, and needs originate from the interaction of one individual with another; (2) anxiety is the chief disruptive force in interpersonal relationships—the need for relief of anxiety is the need for interpersonal security; and (3) individuals may distort present day relationships by projecting expectations as a result of former relationships—it is the role of the therapeutic agent to enable individuals to evaluate and obtain feedback about the here and now.

Origin of emotions and behavior in interaction

The principle of the origin of emotions and behavior in the interaction of one individual with another is perhaps the chief principle held by interpersonal theorists and the basis of many group theorists' concentration on the here-and-now interaction of members in groups.

Sullivan's[19] original intention in focusing on the origins of emotions and behavior in light of individuals' interaction was to explain how significant relationships in the past may function to explain present day disabilities in individuals' interaction with others. He focused heavily on the mother-child relationship, but also on the particular patterns of interaction that occur among individuals and their siblings and among individuals and their parents. Sullivan identified the mother-child relationship as the source of anxiety for the child but also as the means of relieving anxiety. Having established that emotions and behavior may have their origins in the interaction of the mother and the child (between individuals), Sullivan and other theorists, such as Frieda Fromm-Reichmann, explored the origins of interpersonal dysfunctioning—emotional illness with respect to the interaction of individuals with one another.

The principle of the origin of emotions and behavior in the interaction of one individual with another in a group setting is currently utilized in two distinctively different ways. In one instance this principle is utilized to examine members' current ways of behaving in respect to former relationships with parental figures. Quite often the intent is personality reconstruction. In a second instance it is utilized to analyze the sequential unfolding of interaction between members in the here and now; insight into how members affect each other is the goal. In both instances, however, the emotions and behavior of a member seems to be a result of his interaction with others and not related to the strength or weakness of his id, ego, or superego.

The goal being personality reconstruction, the leader will consider feelings, thoughts, and behavior arising between two members of the group as clues to similar problems with interpersonal relationships in the past. He may, for example, identify an interchange between himself and another member who was fearful of being punished by the leader as an episode that can only be fully understood if the group examines the nature of this member's previous relationship with parental figures.

The leader should encourage members to relate to the group their relationship with their parents. A good example of this approach is that of Ezriel,[8] who also discussed various groups where the leader relied on this principle to interpret what was going on in the group. Essentially Ezriel delineates the role of transference—the projection of former thoughts and behavior on current figures—in a group setting.

With the goal of developing members' insight into the nature of group interaction in the here and now, the leader will treat individuals' feelings, thoughts, and behavior in an entirely different fashion. Feelings of one member will be analyzed in terms of the behavior of one or more group members, for example. In turn his behavior may be seen to affect others' feelings, and so on. The leader may encourage members to relate their thoughts and feelings one after another in order for the group to get a clearer picture of how they affect and are affected by the others. Instances of one member's feeling angry would be analyzed in terms of his perceptions of others' thoughts or feelings and not in terms of his thoughts and feelings in reference to persons in his past. The leader may never relate the here-and-now interaction of members to their relationships with significant others in similar situations.

Anxiety and interpersonal security

The role of anxiety as the chief disruptive force in interpersonal relationships and the need for interpersonal security is a principle formulated by Sullivan which is directly applicable to group work and the benefits of groups.

Sullivan[19] related early needs for interpersonal security to the infant's dependence on the satisfaction of his biological needs, for example, for food. Since the infant has no capacity for action toward the relief of anxiety, the mother was seen to be his sole source of relief. Later, relief of anxiety, Sullivan thought, was experienced as continued or enhanced self-respect and self-esteem, since relief of anxiety from unsatisfied basic needs was no longer a problem. Sullivan claims that continued or enhanced self-respect and self-esteem is fulfilled by acceptance and prestige founded in interpersonal relationships.

For the purposes of group work, it can be asserted that members' problems in interacting with each other may be viewed in light of their feelings of interpersonal insecurity and their anxiety in relating to others. The basis for relief of this anxiety can be found in the quality of interaction that enhances members' self-esteem and self-respect. The role of the leader is one of developing members' self-esteem and of protecting them from overwhelming feelings of insecurity. The goals the leader sets for the group, the degree of leadership offered in controlling the focus of the group, and even its physical setting may affect members' feelings of security during encounters.

Group theorists, such as Ackerman,[1] Whitaker and Liebermann,[21] and myself, believe that groups may be the ultimate basis of security and esteem for the individual, and therefore a relief from interpersonal insecurity. A problem arises only around creating an environment within the group wherein members feel secure. Many family groups, as well as various reference groups, are great bolsterers of the individual's self-esteem and self-respect.

The problem of members' anxiety due to interpersonal insecurity and members' self-esteem are taken up in depth in Chapter 9, "Introductory Phase," and Chapter 10, case study 4.

Distortion and feedback about current relationships

Sullivan perceived a potential in individuals to selectively ignore present aspects of their relationships with others. He concluded that individuals could live in their own private world, not differentiating between reality and fantasy. Sullivan explains that as long as the individual does not seek validation of his current relationships he can continue to respond to others in light of his distortion. He coined the term *parataxic distortion* to describe the distortion of subsequent opportunities for growth by early anxiety experiences, leading to hindrance of mutual understanding in current interpersonal relationships. Sullivan further concludes that it is the task of the therapeutic relationship to encourage individuals to evaluate the reality of the current relationship and therefore to see their experiences as distortions. If individuals do not evaluate the current situation, present day relationships and interpersonal situations will be misjudged and parataxically distorted along the lines of the individual's unrevised early experiences.

The principle of distortion and need for feedback is directly applicable to an analysis of members' interaction in a group setting. It is possible that these members' responses to one another are based on their expectations from former relationships. In this sense they can be viewed as parataxically distorting the current group situation in light of unrevised earlier experiences with others. One member, for example, may interpret frowns from the leader as signifying rejection and may be fearful of continuing to displease the leader. He decides to stay silent and not risk being ousted by the leader. He makes certain assumptions about the leader's behavior based on his relationships with significant others in the past. Unless he confers with the leader to determine if the leader, in fact, is displeased or unless the leader gives feedback about what he is feeling toward this member, he may continue to distort his relationship with the leader in light of his earlier experiences. As a therapeutic agent the leader should be aware of such possible distortions and should encourage feedback and clarification of members' interpretations of others' feelings, thoughts, and behaviors. By seeking consensual validation around one aspect of interaction or about members' relationships with one another, the group learns what is reality and what it is perceived to be as a result of some members' parataxic distortions.

Communication framework

The basic premises of communication theories developed by Ruesch, Bateson, Jackson, Watzlawick, and Satir have obvious and direct application to the study and practice of group work. In this section we will discuss five propositions put forth by these theorists and relate them to group work. These propositions are (1) communication is inevitable; (2) communication is a multilevel phenomenon; (3) messages contain certain connotations as well as denotations; (4) there are manifest and latent elements in each message sent or received; and (5) when people communicate, they are assuming responsibility for interaction. In discussing these premises, reference will be made to several concepts typically utilized by communication theorists. These concepts will be defined as they appear.

One cannot not communicate

The premise that it is impossible not to communicate is basic to an understanding of communication theory. This premise is based on the assumption that people have an inherent need to communicate their needs and demands, learned to communicate very early in life, and continue to do so whether by words or gestures in order to seek gratification. A great deal of an individual's communication is thought to be nonverbal, such as that expressed in one's facial movements, gestures, posture, and movement toward and away from objects and other persons. Even silence can be a form of communication. Although individuals have the power to decide which mode of communication they will rely on, they cannot not communicate.

In a group setting the leader, as well as the members, should be cognizant of the fact that communication is occurring even if no one is saying anything at the time. Posture, seating arrangements, gestures, and facial expressions communicate information about members to others. Often members are entirely unaware of the fact that others have received messages about their moods, thoughts, of feelings, since they have not revealed them through the use of words. It is the task of the leader to make known to the group that members are communicating through nonverbal, as well as verbal, means and to help them decipher what it is that they are communicating to one another. Ruesch[14] claims that the leader has several tools at his disposal to help decipher messages and improve the quality of group communication: the leader may (1) acknowledge the nonverbal messages people are sending—thereby strengthening individuals' desires to communicate, as well as giving them the initial pleasure of being received; (2) acknowledge with understanding the nonverbal messages; this kind of exchange, although pleasurable for the sender, often leads to misunderstanding, since the sender can easily assume the group has in fact "read" him; and (3) acknowledge without understanding the nonverbal communication in the group; this form of intervention is most fruitful with nonverbal communication or any other messages that seem unclear as it elicits elaboration from members. The leader, by stating that he hears or perceives the member to be communicating but does not quite understand what he intends, indicates to the sender that if he does not elaborate, especially with words, the group has no way of knowing for sure if they have perceived him correctly. When the leader encourages members to check out the meaning of messages as well as the free flow of feedback, he is providing an atmosphere where members can learn and correct errors in communication. The leader can do this more easily if he is able to illustrate and convince the group that they cannot not communicate.

Communication as a multilevel phenomenon

Watzlawick[20] and Satir (and Ruesch to a lesser extent) stress the proposition that communication is a multilevel phenomenon. What Watzlawick means is that there is a content or informational value to messages and to certain of their aspects which explain what the message is about and how the sender conceives of his relationship with the receiver.

For example, the following statement from one member to others in the group illustrates this point.

"If you think I'm going to do all the talking in this group, you're mistaken; I expect other people to talk too."

One aspect of informational value in this message is the expressed expectation of the member: "I expect other people to talk more." An aspect of the message that tells the group how the sender conceives of his relationship with the others is the implied message: "You're making excessive demands on me to do the talking here, and I want it to stop—other members should assume responsibility for the discussion in the group." A third message refers to the feelings the sender has and is told in his tone of voice and choice of words: "I'm angry at you."

The group may choose to look at any aspect of the statement or may ignore that part of the message which describes the relationship of the sender to the group. Since the sender seems to be concerned about his relationship with the group at this point, it would appear that the group would focus on this aspect of the message. Still the fact that there were at least three different messages may confuse the group as to what the sender intended to do through his communication.

If the group is made aware of the fact that messages can have more than one level, that they are made up of information, expressions of feelings, and statements about relationships, members will be able to recognize the complexity of communication in the group. In a group setting, members have the option of considering all aspects of a message; but first they must be aware of the different levels as opposed to taking the communication at face value. Obviously the group cannot possibly dissect each message sent; it must decide which messages to examine more closely and which to let escape further scrutinization. The leader's judgment is most important in this matter. The leader should be fully aware of what he hopes to accomplish by analyzing an aspect of communication and should consider the impact on both individuals who have sent or received the messages and on the group as a whole. The direction the leader sets for the group in choosing what messages to examine and how it is accomplished will determine the therapeutic process for the group and individual members.

Messages connote and denote

The fact that messages, words as well as nonverbal expressions, have connotations as well as denotations make communication highly complex. The resulting problem that arises, as explained by Watzlawick,[20] is that the message sent is not necessarily the message received. Essentially, what the sender intends to denote by his message does not necessarily have the same connotation for others. The following example may further illustrate this fact.

"Well, I guess you could say that my life hasn't been 'a bowl of cherries.'"

What the sender means by this statement is not entirely clear. The message may be intended to denote something very specific; yet it could connote different things to various people. To one person it might connote that his life has not been easy at times. To another his message may be interpreted as meaning that his life has not always been colorful and exciting, or that his life has been difficult because he was hurt many times. Since messages can denote and connote different things, they can easily be misunderstood. If no one bothers to evaluate what the sender actually meant to denote, the sender will most likely continue to be misunderstood.

The implications of this principle for group work are somewhat obvious. In a group setting where members are sending and receiving messages, it is possible that they will be misunderstood or will misunderstand others because their messages may be interpreted in several ways. It is important for group members to be made aware of the fact that the message they send might not be the message received by others in the group. The leader can be instrumental in pointing this out. By asking for different interpretations of an unclear message, members learn the complexities of their communications from the incongruency of others' perceptions. This procedure will point out that messages connote different things to different persons. As a result, members are more apt to clarify their statements and check out how they have been received.

Manifest and latent elements of communication

Closely related to the proposition that communication is a multilevel phenomenon is the premise that all communication has manifest and latent elements. By manifest we mean the overt message, which may be feelings, thoughts, or opinions that the sender is aware of and is purposely revealing in his communication. Latent elements, on the other hand, refer to hidden or covert aspects of communication that the sender is not aware of and has little control over when communicating with others. These latent aspects may also be feelings or thoughts that the sender is *not* aware of but which he gives clues about during interaction with others. Thoughts or feelings may be communicated through his tone of voice, choice of words, facial expression, or the timing of his silence.

Using the following communication, we can hypothesize as to the latent and manifest aspects of the messages sent.

Insincerely stated, "Gee, did what I say hurt you; I'm sorry." And the sender smiles at the receiver.

At first glance we could conclude from the overt message sent that the sender is sorry that he hurt the receiver. However, there is something about the sender's tone of voice and smile that makes us think there is more substance to his feelings than that which is expressed openly. We have clues from his tone of voice and facial expression that he is not altogether sorry or that he may even be glad that he hurt the other person. Most likely these feelings are not completely known to the sender. In fact he may deny them altogether because he has no awareness of them. He may also be unaware of the fact that he is sending this double message. We call the feelings of gladness and the means by which they are communicated the latent elements of this communication.

In a group setting there will be several opportunities to examine both latent and manifest elements of members' communication. The leader can direct the group in this process, as well as determine the extent to which it deals with latent aspects of messages. Pointing out the possibility of double messages is one approach to teaching the group about these aspects of communication.

Responsibility in communicating

Finally the premise discussed by Satir[15] that when one communicates he accepts responsibility for the interaction, leads us to consider the whole area of what is meant by functional or dysfunctional communication. Satir suggests that when individuals cannot assume responsibility for interaction that ensues, their communication becomes dysfunctional. For example, the communicator may deliver conflicting messages, act on assumption, leave out whole connections, or act as if he communicated when in fact he did not. Dysfunctional communication is a result of failure in learning to communicate properly, as well as the inability of the communicator to accept the responsibility of communicating with others.

The following example from a group illustrates dysfunctional communication. One member is angry with the leader for not directing the group as the member thinks it should be. He does not complete his message that he is angry at the leader because he cannot take the responsibility for his feelings, since he fears they will evoke retaliation. He may also be unable to accept the fact that he can be destructive in his relationships with others and therefore will block out of his awareness any negative feelings that he may have toward the leader or any other member in the group. If he communicates clearly, he not only must take the responsibility for what he provokes but also must recognize unacceptable features about himself. Faced with these consequences he may choose dysfunctional communication and avoid responsibility for what he may have communicated.

The leader should be aware of the fact that dysfunctional communication serves a purpose for group members. When he points out dysfunctional patterns he may force members to become more responsible for their interactions in the group, and this may be quite threatening. Members will need support and a sense of security if they are to look at and change their dysfunctional patterns. The leader's treatment of the dysfunctional communicator, timing, and the participation of other group members is terribly important if he is to move him toward more effective communication. Direct confrontation is not always helpful. Satir[15] recommends that a good portion of the leader's role should involve acting as a model communicator. Otherwise the leader should communicate clearly and directly. By pointing out discrepancies, spelling out nonverbal communication, and identifying double messages, the leader can help others learn to communicate clearly and directly. However, this should be done in an environment free of threat. In essence, then, the leader acts as a model communicator and builds up members' self-esteem as he helps them establish more effective modes of communication.

Case study 1, "Dysfunctional Communication Syndromes in a Married Couples Group," discusses the concept of dysfunctional communication and how leaders can intervene effectively with this phenomena.

Group dynamics and group process framework

An area contributing much to the study and practice of group work is the theory of group dynamics and group process that has been developed since 1940 by Bonner, Cartwright, and Zander; Luft, Knowles, and Knowles; Bradford, Whitaker, and Liebermann; and many others. The propositions discussed here are those basic to a theory of group dynamics and group process. These include (1) groups are in a constant state of flux; (2) the movement of groups is discernible and can be described as stages or phases of group development; the phases and stages of group development depend on the extent to which groups have resolved members' concerns about intimacy and authority; and (3) groups have the potential to develop along healthy lines or may resort to unhealthy adaptation, depending on opportunities within the group to successfully resolve problems or concerns.

Groups are in a constant state of flux

Bonner,[7] Bennis and Shepard,[2] Whitaker and Liebermann[21] and other group process theorists view groups to be in a constant state of flux. Bonner and Whitaker and Liebermann conceive the group and events that occur in terms of an equilibrium model. Bonner claims that groups whose members interact in a changing and adjusting relationship are always attempting to restore equilibrium within the group. Essentially individuals are in a state of tension in respect to others in the group and seek a resolution of these tensions in an attempt to return to a new level of homeostasis. Whitaker and Liebermann claim that even within single group sessions, at any given moment the group situation can be understood in terms of forces toward equilibrium, that is, that the group's movement within the session can be seen as successive shifts in equilibrium.

To summarize, groups can be conceived not only as static, unchanging aggregates of individuals but as individuals interacting in response to group tensions in an attempt to reduce these tensions. The process or movement within groups relates to members interacting in response to and for the reduction of tensions occurring within the group. These tensions arise from the unique interaction among members and must be reduced if the group is to remain intact. The movement of the group in reference to these tensions indicates an attempt to restore homeostasis.

The fact that groups are not static cautions us to be aware that although we are concerned with present conditions, we must also analyze this state in terms of what has occurred before and what will evolve. Bonner and Whitaker and Liebermann, for example, consider that group norms arise from members' interaction and undergo revision until they are crystallized as part of the group culture. A norm, such as expressing one's personal problems within the group, arises from the needs of its members. Through the interaction of members in reference to fears and opposing forces, this norm may undergo complete or partial revision before it is finally crystallized. The resulting norm may be to express only those problems that the group can handle or share with other members.

The premise of group movement can determine the role of the leader. If the leader is aware that groups are constantly shifting in reference to tensions, he will realize the necessity of depicting certain phases of the group in respect to the resolution of these tensions. He will need to know what these tensions are and how they determine the behavior, feelings, and thoughts of members, as well as changes in behavior. He will not attribute the interaction of group members to individuals' personalities but will visualize it in terms of group movement toward and away from common tensions. For example, the action of members to deny that the group needs help from the leader would not be analyzed in terms of individual personalities but as an indication that the group as a whole is responding to an issue about its own dependence in respect to authority relations. Necessarily the leader will encourage members to become aware of the interaction of the group in terms of total group movement rather than in manifestations of individual personalities. The leader would stop the group and ask members questions about what has happened in the session thus far, how it compares with what has happened in previous sessions, and what meaning it has for the group remaining intact.

Movement of the group in stages or phases

Having asserted that groups are in a constant state of flux and having suggested that their movement may be discernible as phases or stages of development, we will discuss the movement more specifically. Rather than simply categorizing the phases of group movement as introductory, established, and termination, some group theorists (Bennis and Shepard[2] and Schutz[17]) have attempted to identify group phases or stages according to the resolution of common group tensions. Although these theorists differ in the titles they assign to group phases, they concur that these stages reflect members' responses to the issues of intimacy and authority within the group. Whitaker and Liebermann[21] suggest that members enter the group with expectations of what a group will do for them; within the group they are faced with competition and the reality of how certain expectations are treated. The orderliness that occurs within the group in respect to these problems can be conceptualized in terms of a continuous problem-solving process around intimacy and authority.

Bennis and Shepard,[2] in describing phases of T-group development, identify dependence and interdependence as the major issues of internal uncertainty common to and important in all groups. Dependency relates to the orientation toward the handling and distribution of power; interdependence, to members' feelings about closeness with others. Bennis and Shepard describe the group as it moves from phase I, dependence, through phase II, interdependence. Within each phase they identify several subphases, which describe more specifically the reaction of the group in respect to these issues, for example, *phase I* (1) dependence—flight, (2) counterdependence—fight, and (3) resolution—catharsis; *phase II* (4) enchantment—flight, (5) disenchantment—fight, and (6) consensual validation.

In this analysis of group phases and stages of development, Schutz[6] relates phases of group development to the establishment and maintenance of relations between members in reference to certain interpersonal needs, such as intimacy and control. He explains that to function effectively the group must find a comfortable balance in regard to the amount of contact members have with each other, control and influence, and personal closeness. He conceptualizes three issues of group development usually taken up by the group in this sequence—inclusion, control, and affection. In the initial sessions Schutz maintains that members need to feel included and to include others. Fulfillment of these needs usually comprises the beginning activity of the group. Members also need to influence others and to be influenced if the group is to make decisions. Without such influence, no decision-making system can be effective. During the working phase of the group, members must be preoccupied with the issue of who will control or direct the group and to what extent others will share in the control. Finally, members need to express and receive affection. Not only is it required that individuals relate to each other with sufficient warmth and closeness for group processes to proceed; but at certain points, expression of warmth and affection is appropriate. At termination, for example, members are usually evaluating the growth of the group and are occupied with warmth and close feelings toward the group as a whole and toward certain members in particular.

A final mode of categorizing phases of group development is to examine the general issues of intimacy and authority in reference to the concept of common group tensions or conflicts as is characteristic of the theories of Ezriel[8] and Whitaker and Liebermann.[21] Ezriel and Whitaker and Liebermann examine the wishes, fears, and solutions involved in the issues of intimacy and authority. The phases of the group in terms of the theories relate to the group's movement toward expressing certain wishes, eliminating its fears, and thereby evolving enabling solutions that operate to move the group forward to a new level of equilibrium. The focal conflict model of group development is presented in the psychoanalytic framework—the existence of unconscious motives (pp. 88-89); the reader is encouraged to review this discussion.

Healthy and unhealthy group development

How the flux and movement of group dynamics may result in healthy or unhealthy group adaptation is the subject of this discussion. First, however, it is important to clarify what is meant by healthy or unhealthy adaptation. According to Schutz's[16] theory of interpersonal needs, if the group has maintained a viable level of closeness and a process of control over its members so that effective decision making results, then we may categorize the group as having achieved healthy adaptation. If the group has not met members' needs for inclusion and intimacy, or if members cannot influence each other or have established patterns of overcontrol, then we would conclude that a state of unhealthy adaptation exists.

Whitaker and Liebermann[21] give us additional suggestions about defining group movement as healthy or unhealthy. They suggest that the development of the group from inception to termination is characterized by the recurrence of common group concerns and that what ensues should be progressively expanding cultural conditions to allow members to deal more successfully with these issues. Bennis and Shepard[2] explain that until the group meets with some success in these major areas of internal uncertainty or in overcoming other obstacles to valid communication, anxieties in other areas cannot be reduced. If the group is unable to resolve its anxieties concerning dependency or interdependency, it forestalls its abilities to solve problems in other areas of group life and, in one sense, becomes ineffectual. This can occur particularly if there are no conflict-free members to assist in reducing the uncertainty characterizing a given phase or if the leader does not act as a catalyst to reduce uncertainty.

It is not, then, that groups are destined toward either a healthy or unhealthy adaptation but that the group's formation along either line requires successful resolution of specific group concerns—namely, those regarding issues of authority and intimacy. Without the aid of unconflicted group members or a leader who can act as a catalyst in the group to reduce uncertainty, there is little likelihood of resolution and healthy adaptation.

It is the task of the group leader not only to distinguish between healthy and unhealthy group formation but also to intervene and produce resolution of issues and healthy adaptation. He must mobilize and utilize the conflict-free capacity of the group. He can choose interventions that would enable members to achieve successful solutions to group conflicts about authority and intimacy; for example, he can help members identify their concerns about getting close to one another, thereby reducing their anxieties of impending intimacy with each other. The leader can help the group become aware of how members manifest certain concerns, such as their need for structure and to feel included, and can put these concerns in perspective in light of ongoing group development. Such awareness will also reduce members' anxieties about intimacy and authority, since members are able to understand that the issues and concerns with which they are confronted confront all groups and that they are not unusual in their reactions to these issues. The leader, as a rule, can do much to guide the group toward a healthy adaptation. He needs, however, to be aware of common tensions that arise around the issues of intimacy and authority and of how they are manifested in the group. The leader must also have certain skills in mobilizing the conflict-free capacity of the group, as well as in intervening to enable the group to achieve successful solutions for these issues.

Existential and Gestalt frameworks

Thus far several theories have been taken up independently; certain premises from psychoanalytic, interpersonal, communication, and group dynamics theories have been discussed. Now two additional theoretical frameworks that greatly influence contemporary approaches to group work and that have certain premises in common will be considered. They share to some extent the beliefs that (1) man is free to define himself and cultivate his unique individuality within certain limitations; (2) the nature of becoming lies in the individual's awareness of the here and now and his capacity for change; and (3) people can deal adequately with their own life problems if they know *what* they are and not necessarily *why* they exist. These propositions are found to pervade the philosophies of group leaders who deal solely with the here and now and who provide members an experience in becoming more aware of the feelings they have suppressed due to their own personal constraints or expectations of others in the society at large.

Freedom to cultivate one's individuality

Perls,[13] Maslow,[11] and May[12] adhere to the principle that man is free to cultivate his own unique individuality. They believe that man has a basic need to be understood as a unique person and to find out what he is, what satisfies him, and what he wants and that he must allow himself to achieve self-actualization. Since man is free to define himself, he has no alibi for insisting that he has no freedom. His limits are areas in which he is fearful or feels pain; yet growth in these areas is rewarding. Inherent in this philosophical premise is that man must at all times assume responsibility for himself; no one else can do this for him. From the viewpoint of these Gestalt and existential theorists, if individuals are free to cultivate their own individuality, they are never without a choice about how they feel, think, and behave.

In a group setting, members are not always aware of their full potential to choose one of several ways of feeling, thinking, and behaving. In addition they frequently claim that their emotions and behavior are out of the realm of their control. Through increased awareness of alternatives displayed by other members, as well as through increased awareness of the variety of feelings, thoughts, and behaviors they themselves display, members become more fully cognizant of the choices open to them.

It is the task of the leader to point out to members that they are never without a choice as to how they feel, think, and behave and that they employ this deception to avoid total responsibility for themselves. The leader may point out that the reason why members may blame others for their hostile behavior is that they cannot accept this aspect of themselves. But they also point out that knowing oneself as potentially hostile is a part of knowing oneself as a unique individual who is capable of a variety of feelings and behavior, no matter how undesirable these may appear. The group as a whole can aid individuals in discovering the self if it encourages members to be aware of all aspects. Members' acceptance of experimentation and encouragement to get in touch with feelings, thoughts, and behavior are important if they are to explore their unique individuality in the group. Feedback to one another provides them with necessary information about how they will be received when they assume full responsibility for their being.

Nature of becoming in awareness of the here and now

To the existentialist an individual's own experience is his highest authority on what he is and what he can be. If individuals are fully present in the immediacy of the moment and if they are open to all aspects of their being, they are able to transcend themselves and develop their potentialities. To the Gestalt theorist, if individuals are in full contact with the here and now of what they are thinking, feeling, and how they are behaving, they are in fact accepting and integrating all aspects of the self. If individuals accept and integrate all aspects of the self (the "good" and the "bad" me, for example) they are able to experience more fully what it is to be what they are, and their ability to be creative is not inhibited.

The premise that the nature of becoming is in the awareness of the here and now can direct much of the activity that occurs in groups led by existential and Gestalt leaders. Members are encouraged to relate their feelings, thoughts, and behavior to what is happening in the here and now. The group spends little time on what has happened in previous sessions or on what members have experienced in relationships in the past, since the leader believes that a knowledge of the here and now, not a knowledge of the past, frees members to change and achieve greater self-actualization. Usually group members are asked to take turns in relating their feelings and thoughts in sequence. Member 1 may relate in the following manner: "I am feeling scared; I am experiencing the scaredness in my hands; I am aware of my hands shaking; I wish they would stop; I can see everybody staring at me; I feel very uncomfortable; (pause) I am less uncomfortable now, but I still want to stop; I am stopping." Member 1 had an opportunity through this exercise to become more completely aware of what happens to him in the group—what his feelings are, how he experiences his feelings, how he relates them to what he perceives in the group, and what alternatives are open to him, for example, to stop or continue feeling what he is feeling. The assumption that Gestalt and existential theorists make in reference to this increased awareness is that once member 1 became aware of his experiences, he had an opportunity to transcend himself and choose an alternative, for example, to stop talking, an alternative which may not have been clear to him otherwise. If member 1 did not have an opportunity to explore this fear in this manner, presumably he would not have been aware of alternatives open to him and would have gone on feeling scared, or would have associated change in his feelings with what goes on in the group, external to himself. For example, the *group* is making me anxious.

Dealing adequately knowing what, not why

Closely related to the first two propositions is the idea that people can deal adequately with their own life problems if they know *what* these problems are and not necessarily *why* they exist. This principle borders on both the premise that man is free to define himself and that his freedom depends on his awareness of the here and now. Basically, if man knows what his problems are, through his awareness of his limitations in the here and now, he can sufficiently deal with them himself. What is implied here is that dealing with problems is a growth process, not a corrective process. The self needs to be expanded through increased self-actualization (knowing what), not corrected through discipline, retraining, or discovery of underlying motives (knowing why).

The idea that people can deal adequately with their own life problems, if they know what they are, is an additional rationale for the leader of the group to keep members focused on the here and now of their experience in the group. By focusing on the here and now, members are sufficiently diverted from examining "why" and are, at the same time, totally preoccupied with "what." If they are totally absorbed with "what," they are also less likely to project, deny, or desensitize themselves to their feelings and thoughts. Thus they are more likely to become fully present in the immediacy of the situation and therefore more aware of alternatives in respect to solutions for their problems.

The overall goals of the leader relate to his belief that individuals need to identify with and accept the forming self. If they do not, their ability to be creative and handle their own life problems is inhibited. It is the purpose of the group experience to provide an environment for individuals to identify with and accept the forming self through experiences of awareness, until this sense of self is revised to the point that oneself ("I") is the one thinking, perceiving, feeling, and doing.

Behavioral modification framework

A final theoretical orientation influencing the nature of group work, and which can be extremely useful to the nurse, is behavior modification. Behavior therapy in psychiatry has been quite influential in group and individual treatment approaches, especially in group therapy with children. Children with developmental disabilities and children with emotional disorders who do not readily respond to psychoanalytic techniques, nor appreciate self-awareness measures, can be treated successfully with the use of behavior modification techniques in small groups. The origin of this theory dates back to the work of Pavlov, Skinner,[23] and others who concerned themselves with theories of conditioning behavior. The initial intent was to present a practical alternative to a theory such as Freudian analysis, which focuses on the "why." Like existential and Gestalt theories, behavior modification focuses on "what"—that is, the specific behaviors that present themselves in the here and now. It does not explore the basis of the behavior in the unconscious operations of the mind. It does, however, stress tangible motivation in the form of reinforcers to influence a change in behavior.

The concepts and principles that are relevant for group work and that are selected for discussion include the following:

1. Behaviors are adaptive or maladaptive.
2. Behavior change results from external positive or negative reinforcement.
3. Social climate of group has impact on behavior.
4. Behavior change is measurable.

Behaviors are adaptive or maladaptive

Unlike other personality theories that pinpoint individual deficiencies in terms of a weak ego, weak personality, or disease process affecting total systems of the body, behavioral theorists choose to see specific behaviors as adaptive or maladaptive. Hostile attacks, hyperactivity, "crazy" behavior, and undesirable or unhealthy habits (for example, depriving oneself of food [the anorexic], drinking excessively [the alcoholic] or compulsive hand washing [compulsive neurosis] are deemed maladaptive or undesirable because they prevent the individual from functioning adequately in his environment. As maladaptive behaviors they are the targets for the change, not the underlying personality structure itself. Target behaviors are the symptoms that the individual and group leader work to modify during the course of a goal-oriented program. The program clearly establishes the desired change expected and how it will be achieved.

For example, a program for an entire group may be established to increase verbal exchange around a central theme, for example, how you feel about your siblings. The target behaviors in the group would be members' punching, teasing, and interrupting others when they are talking about their feelings about their sisters and brothers. The group is told and shown that listening and talking about the subject will earn them a "happy face" decal at 5-minute intervals in the group. The target behaviors will elicit dismissal consequences from the group if three or more episodes of punching, teasing, or interrupting occur during the group session.

Members are aware (1) that it is their behavior that is the focus and (2) what the target or maladaptive behaviors are, as well as (3) how their target behavior will be treated in the group.

Behavior change results from external positive or negative reinforcement

Integral to the behavior modification framework is the premise that behavior change results from punishment of undesirable acts or positive reinforcement of desirable alternative behaviors. Rewarding behavior such as giving children happy faces depends on knowing what the child values and would like for himself. Rewards based on others' values, and which are not seen to be desirable to the patient, are irrelevant behavior reinforcers for that individual and will not produce a behavior change. Likewise, for reinforcement to be viewed as negative it must be seen by the specific child to elicit undesirable consequences.

Tokens or objects that can be accumulated and later exchanged for material and social positive reinforcers indirectly connote rewards to the child. Poker chips and stars, for example, when accumulated, could be exchanged for privileges that the child desires; this is referred to as a token system of reinforcement.

Reinforcement of changes over a period of time is felt to increase desired acts and decrease adherence to destructive and maladaptive patterns. The more immediately a behavior is reinforced, the more effectively will its strength be changed by the reinforcement.

Social climate of group has impact on behavior

A group setting for behavior change involves two interrelating principles. Group membership can be seen by members to be a reinforcer. Membership promotes feelings of belonging and interactions where one can be heard and appreciated by others. In itself, group membership is a source of positive social reinforcement where belonging and being able to go to group meetings can serve as a reward to members. In this case, dismissal from the group is also a punishment.

Likewise, the way members and the leader respond to an individual's behavior inside the group may be viewed as reinforcing or punishing. The power of the group to socially induce changes in symptoms, for example, monopolizing, hallucinating, and performing aggressive acts, is a well-known phenomenon and is integrated into the practice and research of other theorists, such as the analytic–group process leaders who study the influence of early group norms on member behavior.

The group then serves as an environment for behavior change in two distinct ways: (1) membership can connote a reward in itself—if it bestows status to the individual—and (2) group feedback can further influence target behaviors as they are acted out in the sessions.

Behavior change is measurable

The concept that behavior changes are observable and measurable is still another important principle of this theory. It has direct implication for the establishment of a plan for the group and a program for certain members in a group.

Since behavior change is measurable, we are obligated to know and assess degrees of initial maladaptation and document success in changing individuals or the group as a whole.

Baseline data refers to the accumulation of information that allows us to make a quantitative statement about the level of maladaptation. If we are making statements about all group members, we can specify how many display the target behaviors how often. If we focus on an individual member, we can specify how often he displays the target behaviors.

If we monitor, measure, and count target behaviors over time, beginning with operant level measurements, continuing during periods of the group when reinforcement is used, we can judge the effects of the behavior modification program on the extinction of target behaviors. This principle of measuring concrete aspects of change is an evaluation concept that has applicability for other group treatment approaches but is utilized uniquely by the behavioral modification theorist as a basis for intervention as well as research.

In conclusion the nurse who integrates the behavior modification framework in his group work will

1. Identify target behaviors
2. Establish a baseline measurement of the target behavior
3. Identify appropriate positive and negative reinforcers given the individual child or group value system as a whole
4. Formulate and apply a consistent plan for rewarding desired changes
5. Monitor and measure alterations in the target behavior

The nurse will appreciate the fact that the group itself can be viewed as a social reinforcement and utilize this premise in analyzing behavior changes in the group.

REFERENCES

1. Ackerman, N. W.: Introduction processes in a group and the role of the leader, Psychoanal. Soc. Sci. **4:**111-120, 1955.
2. Bennis, W. G., and Shepard, H. A.: A theory of group development, Hum. Rel. **9:**415-457, 1956.
3. Berne, E.: Principles of group treatment, New York, 1969, Grove Press.
4. Berne, E.: A layman's guide to psychiatry and psycho-analysis, ed. 2, New York, 1968, Simon & Schuster.
5. Berne, E.: Transactional analysis in psychotherapy, New York, 1961, Grove Press.
6. Biernoff, J.: Lectures in psychoanalysis, University of California School of Nursing, University of California Medical Center, San Francisco, fall-spring quarters, 1966-1967.
7. Bonner, H.: Group dynamics—principles and applications, New York, 1964, The Ronald Press Co.

8. Ezriel, H.: The role of transference in psycho-analytic and other approaches to group treatment, Acta Psychother. **7:**101-116, 1959.
9. Ezriel, H.: A psychoanalytic approach to group treatment, Br. J. Med. Psychol. **23:**59-74, 1950.
10. Freud, S.: A general introduction to psychoanalysis, New York, 1924, Washington Square Press.
11. Maslow, A. H.: Toward a psychology of being, Princeton, N.J., 1962, D. Van Nostrand Co.
12. May, R., editor: Existential psychology, New York, 1961, Random House.
13. Perls, F., Hefferline, R., and Goodman, P.: Gestalt therapy, New York, 1951, Julian Press.
14. Ruesch, J.: Therapeutic communication, New York, 1961, W. W. Norton & Co.
15. Satir, V. M.: Conjoint family therapy—a guide to theory and technique, Palo Alto, Calif., 1964, Science and Behavior Books.
16. Schutz, W.: Interpersonal underworld (reprint), New York, 1968, Holt, Rinehart & Winston.
17. Schutz, W.: The ego, FIRO theory and the leader as completer (reprint), New York, 1968, Holt, Rinehart & Winston.
18. Skinner, B. F.: Science and human behavior, New York, 1953, The Macmillan Co.
19. Slavson, S. R.: A textbook in analytic group psychotherapy, New York, 1964, Columbia University Press.
20. Sullivan, H. S.: The interpersonal theory of psychiatry, New York, 1953, W. W. Norton & Co.
21. Watzlawick, P.: An anthology of human communication, Palo Alto, Calif., 1964, Science & Behavior Books, Inc.
22. Whitaker, D. S., and Liebermann, M. A.: Psychotherapy through the group process, New York, 1964, Atherton Press.
23. Wolfe, A., and Schwartz, E. K.: Psychoanalysis in groups, New York, 1962, Grune & Stratton.

SUGGESTED READINGS
Introduction

Durkin, H.: The development of systems theory and its implications for the theory and practice of group therapy. In Wolberg, L., and Aronson, M., editors: Group therapy 1975, New York, 1975, Stratton Intercontinental Medical Bank Corp.
Lieberman, M.: Group therapies. In Usden, G., editor: Overview of psychotherapies, New York, 1975, Brunner/Mazel.
Naar, R.: A theoretical framework for group psychotherapy, J. Contemp. Psychother. **7:**50-55, 1975.
Surim, R., and Weigel, R., editors: The innovative psychological therapies: critical and creative contributions, New York, 1975, Harper & Row, Publishers.

Psychoanalytic framework

Akerman, N. W.: Psychoanalysis and group psychotherapy, J. Sociopsychopathol. Soc. **3:** 204-215, 1950.
Brill, A. A.: Basic principles of psychoanalysis, New York, 1949, Doubleday & Co.
Ezriel, H.: The role of transference in psychoanalytic and other approaches to group treatment, Acta Psychoter. **7:**101-116, 1959.
Foulkes, S. H.: Group analytic dynamics with specific reference to psychoanalytic concepts, Int. J. Group Psychother. **2:**1-15, 1961.
Foulkes, S. H., and Anthony, E. J.: Group psychotherapy—the psychoanalytic approach, Baltimore, 1957, Penguin Books.
Foulkes, S.: On groups—analytic psychotherapy. In Rosenbaum, M. and Berger, M.: Group psychotherapy and group function, ed. 2, New York, 1975, Basic Books, Inc., Publishers.

Freud, S.: Group psychology and the analysis of the ego, New York, 1960, Bantam Books.

King, P.: Life cycle—in the Tavistock study group, Perspect. Psychiatr. Care **8:**180-184, 1975.

Lock, N.: Group psychoanalysis: theory and technique, New York, 1961, New York University Press.

Riosch, M.: The work of Wilfred Bion on groups, Psychiatry **33:**56-66, 1970.

Sandner, D.: Bion's analytic theory of groups and its relation to group psychotherapy and group dynamics, Gruppenpsychotherapy Gruppendynamic **9:**1-17, 1975.

Scheidlinger, S.: Psychoanalysis and group behavior, New York, 1952, W. W. Norton & Co.

Wolb, A.: Psychoanalysis in groups. In Rosenbaum, M., and Berger, M., editors: Group psychotherapy and group function, ed. 2, New York, 1975, Basic Books, Inc., Publishers.

Interpersonal framework

Burton, G.: Personal, impersonal and interpersonal relations, New York, 1964, Springer Publishing Co.

Geller, J. J.: Parataxic distortions in the initial stages of group relationships, Int. J. Group Psychother. **12:**27-34, 1962.

Hall, C. S., and Lindzey, G.: Theories of personality, New York, 1957, John Wiley & Sons.

Leary, T.: Interpersonal diagnosis of personality, New York, 1957, The Ronald Press Co.

Lewin, K.: A dynamic theory of personality, New York, 1935, McGraw-Hill Book Co.

Mullahy, P.: Contributions of Harry Stack Sullivan, New York, 1952, Heritage Press.

Rogers, C. R.: Counseling and psychotherapy, Boston, 1942, Houghton Mifflin Co.

Stock, D.: Interpersonal concerns during the early sessions of therapy groups, Int. J. Group Psychother. **12:**14-26, 1962.

Sullivan, H. S.: Conceptions of modern psychiatry, New York, 1953, W. W. Norton & Co.

Sullivan, H. S.: The theory of anxiety and the nature of psychotherapy, Am. J. Psychiatry **12:** 3-12, 1949.

Sullivan, H. S.: Introduction to the study of interpersonal relations, Psychiatry **1:**121-134, 1938.

Communication framework

Barnlund, D. C., editor: Interpersonal communications: survey and studies, Palo Alto, Calif., 1968, Houghton Mifflin Co.

Giffin, K., and Patton, B. R.: Basic readings in interpersonal communication, New York, 1971, Harper & Row, Publishers.

Hall, E. T.: The silent language, New York, 1959, Doubleday & Co.

Meerloo, J. A. M.: Conversation and communication, New York, 1952, International Universities Press.

Reusch, J.: Nonverbal communication, Berkeley and Los Angeles, 1956, University of California Press.

Watzlawick, P., Beavin, J., and Jackson, D.: Pragmatics of human communication, New York, 1967, W. W. Norton & Co.

Group dynamics and group process framework

Benne, K., et al.: The laboratory method of changing and learning: theory and application, Palo Alto, Calif., 1975, Science & Behavior Books.

Bradford, L. P., et al.: T-group theory and laboratory method, New York, 1964, John Wiley & Sons.

Cartwright, D., and Zander, A.: Group dynamics, ed. 3, Evanston, Ill., 1968, Row, Peterson & Co.

Cooper, C., editor: Theories of group processes, London, 1975, John Wiley & Sons.

Foulkes, S. H.: Group process and the individual in the therapeutic group, Br. J. Med. Psychol. **34:**23-31, 1961.

Durkin, H.: Toward a common basis for group dynamics, Int. J. Group Psychother. **7:**115-130, 1957.

Knowles, M., and Knowles, H.: Introduction to group dynamics, New York, 1969, Association Press.

Lippit, R., Watson, J., and Westley, B.: The dynamics of planned change, New York, 1958, Harcourt Brace & Co.

Luft, J.: Group processes: an introduction to group dynamics, Palo Alto, Calif., 1963, National Press Books.

Martin, E. A., and Hill, W. F.: Toward a theory of group development, Int. J. Group Psychother. **7:**20-30, 1957.

McDougall, W.: The group mind, New York, 1920, G. P. Putnam's Sons.

Scheidlinger, S.: Group process in group psychotherapy, Am. J. Psychother. **14:**104-120, 346, 363, 1960.

Existential and Gestalt frameworks

Allport, G.: Becoming, New Haven, Conn., 1955, Yale University Press.

Balogh, P.: New ways of getting more real: or does the encounter culture herald the end of psychoanalysis, Int. J. Soc. Psychiatry **21:**126-129, 1975.

Buber, M.: I and thou, Edinburgh, 1937, T. and T. Clark.

Foulds, M.: The experiential—Gestalt growth group experience. In Quinn, R., and Weigh, R., editors: The innovative psychological therapies: critical and creative contributions, New York, 1975, Harper & Row, Publishers.

Harness, L.: The existential use of the self, Am. J. Psychiatry **131:**1-10, 1974.

Jung, C. G.: The undiscovered self, London, 1958, Routledge & Kegan Paul.

May, R., Angel, E., and Ellenberger, H., editors: Existence: a new dimension in psychiatry and psychology, New York, 1958, Basic Books, Inc., Publishers.

Perls, F. S.: The Gestalt therapy, New York, 1956, Julian Press.

Rogers, C. A.: On becoming a person, Boston, 1961, Houghton Mifflin Co.

Sartre, J. P.: Existential psychoanalysis, Chicago, 1953, Henry Regnery Co.

Behavior modification framework

Birk, L.: Intensive group therapy: an effective behavioral-psychoanalytic method, Am. J. Psychiatry **131:**11-17, 1974.

Field, G.: Group assertive training: training for severely disturbed patients, J. Behav. Ther. Exp. Psychiatry **6:**129-134, 1974.

Liberman, R.: Behavioral methods in group and family therapy. In Rosenbaum, M., and Berger, M., editors: Group psychotherapy and group functions, ed. 2, New York, 1975, Basic Books, Inc., Publishers.

LeBow, M.: Behavior modification—a significant method in nursing practice, Englewood Cliffs, N.J., 1973, Prentice-Hall.

Pratt, S., and Fischer, J.: Behavior modification: changing hyperactive behavior in a children's group, Perspect. Psychiatr. Care **13:**37-42, 1975.

Rinn, R., et al.: Training parents of behaviorally disordered children in groups: a three-year program evaluation, Behav. Ther. **6:**378-387, 1975.

Rosenbaum, A., et al.: Behavioral intervention with hyperactive children: group consequences as a supplement to individual contingencies, Behav. Ther. **6:**315, 323, 1975.

Shaffer, J., and Galinsky, M.: Behavior therapy in groups. In Models of group therapy and sensitivity training, Englewood Cliffs, N.J., 1974, Prentice-Hall, pp. 148-164.

Thoresen, C., and Porter, B.: Behavioral group counseling. In Gazda, G., editor: Basic approaches to group psychotherapy and group counseling, Springfield, Ill., 1975, Charles C Thomas, Publisher.

CHAPTER 7

An eclectic theoretical orientation

Introduction

An alternative to espousing one or another of the theories described thus far is to formulate an eclectic theoretical orientation to one's study and practice of group work. That is, one has the option of selecting principles, concepts, and premises from a variety of theories that appear suitable.

For example, in my own use of a theoretical framework, I generally select a combination of principles from the various theories presented in Chapter 6. I adhere to such premises as the existence of unconscious conflicts in a group, the reenactment of the past in present relationships (analysis concepts), origins of emotions and behavior in interaction, anxiety and interpersonal insecurity (interpersonal concepts), communication as a multilevel phenomena, manifest and latent elements of communication, and responsibility in communicating (communication concepts). I also integrate such ideas as group movement in phases and stages (group dynamics concept), the nature of becoming in an awareness of the here and now (existential and Gestalt frameworks), and the group as a context for social reinforcement (behavior modification concept) into my orientation to group work. Although it is not always evident from my analyses of group process that my approach is eclectic, I am able to draw more heavily on any one of these concepts (and their associated frameworks) when it seems relevant.

As Coleman and Broen[1] explain it, the great majority of therapists are eclectic, attempting to be flexible, utilizing concepts and procedures best suited to the given individual or group. According to Wiener,[5] eclectic therapists appear more likely than others to try out enlightened or hopeful new ways and may act as a filter for society, screening out pretentious or wildly unscientific methods that do no practical good.

In this chapter the fallacy of a unidimensional approach will be discussed. Several examples of theories that are, in fact, more eclectic than pure and circumscribed in nature will be given. The basic features of an eclectic orientation will be discussed, and the advantages and disadvantages of these features will be pointed out. Finally the reasons why an eclectic approach may be more suited to the nurse are given, and certain skills and knowledge that nurses should have if they are to utilize such an orientation in the practice and study of group work will be specified.

It is important to point out here that, although I find that an eclectic orientation offers a great deal of freedom to the practitioner in choosing concepts and principles as he sees fit, I believe some practitioners may feel more comfortable if they master one major theoretical framework before they assume the responsibility of selecting principles and concepts from a variety of theories. Other instructors may hold different opinions, however, and prefer to present the student with a number of theories in order that he is not immediately trapped in respect to his approach to group work. Since I believe this argument also has merit, I am willing to concede that an eclectic orientation is an important option to the beginning practitioner who reads this text, as well as to the more advanced student.

The fallacy of a pure and circumscribed theory

In Chapter 6 we outlined five seemingly distinct theories that can be and are employed in the study and practice of group work. It is important to stress that, although these theoretical frameworks are essentially unidimensional in nature, they are not totally pure and circumscribed. To some extent each has been influenced by other frameworks and overlaps with one or more theoretical orientations. We can illustrate this point by reviewing how the theories we discussed can fall into one or more of the five frameworks we identified.

One of the theories can be seen to be both psychoanalytic and group process oriented. Such a theory is Whitaker and Liebermann's[4] theory of group focal conflicts. It is clear that their focus on underlying wishes and fears of the group converges with the psychoanalytic concept of the existence of unconscious motives. Yet it is also clear that Whitaker and Liebermann employ the concept of focal conflict to describe and explain the overall process and dynamics of the group. They explain that the movement of the group consists of resolution of conflicts around issues of authority and intimacy. The group dynamics theorist characteristically looks at the movement of the group in terms of stages or phases in the resolution of such issues. Since Whitaker and Liebermann combine a psychoanalytic and group process orientation to describe what happens in groups, we would necessarily conclude that their theory is somewhat eclectic; that is, it borrows concepts and principles from more than one theoretical framework.

A theory that seems to combine analytic, interpersonal, and group dynamics or group process principles is Schutz's[3] FIRO theory. Schutz bases his theory on accommodation of interpersonal needs in groups. He claims that group activity is focused on the individual's needs to feel included and include others, to control others and be controlled, as well as to give and receive affection and warmth. Schutz implies that the satisfaction of one's needs, as well as the source of his anxieties, lies in his relationships with others; he is basically interpersonal relationship oriented. We can also see that, although his theory is strongly interpersonal, Schutz has borrowed concepts and principles from group dynamics and psychoanalytic theories. Schutz's concept of a group ego is typically psychoanalytic. The notion that a group has distinct divisions—id, ego, and superego—manifested in different members' roles in the group is borrowed from the psychoanalytic idea of divisions of an individual's mind. The group ego represents that feature of the mind which brings reality to bear on an individual's mind. In addition, Schutz's concept that groups deal in phases with interpersonal needs is typically group dynamics in orientation. It is concerned with groups passing through phases or stages in which passage relies on how the group handles certain common issues.

A theory that seems to relate to an analytic, as well as communicative, framework and that finds its chief origin in the interpersonal school of thought is that of Frieda Fromm-Reichmann.[2] Fromm-Reichmann's theory of parataxic distortion illustrates the point that she combines a focus on psychoanalysis with one on interpersonal concepts and implies an indirect link with communication concepts. The notion of parataxic distortion, or the fact that individuals distort their current relations in terms of early dissociated experiences, assumes a basic psychoanalytic premise that present relationships with others are symbolic reenactments of the past. Fromm-Reichmann's explanation that the power of the therapeutic relationship lies in the fact that individuals can check out what is real and what is distortion in terms of their former relationships indicates the importance she places on therapeutic communication as a corrective process for individuals.

In summary, then, these three examples have shown that theories directly or indirectly applicable to the study and practice of group work are to some extent eclectic in their formulation. The overall conclusion that behavioral theories in general and those utilized in group work in particular are unidimensional is somewhat inaccurate and also misleading. The discussion now turns to the features of an eclectic orientation that combines several theoretical notions as the theorist sees fit. This discussion will lead to enumerating some advantages and disadvantages of an eclectic orientation.

Advantages and disadvantages

A truly eclectic theoretical orientation to the study and practice of group work has at least three features worthy of discussion here. These features can be said to be characteristic of some unidimensional theories as well but are probably more frequently associated with an eclectic approach.

One of the three features is its tendency to present a broad but superficial basis for group work. Since an eclectic orientation borrows from a variety of theoretical frameworks, at will, it does not always supply the theoretical links necessary for an in-depth theory, as might a unidimensional orientation. Essentially the theorist has the freedom to select from a number of theories, quite often without realizing the basic assumptions or philosophical underpinnings associated with the selection of one versus another. Without a clear idea of what governs this selection process, the theoretical framework lacks depth even though it is likely to answer a variety of unrelated questions.

A second feature of an eclectic orientation is that it tends to describe, explain, and predict a greater number of phenomena present in the group than does a more unidimensional orientation. With a unidimensional orientation, for example, one which focuses exclusively on unconscious motives for behavior in the group, one need not necessarily be concerned with describing the group movement through certain phases or the manifestation of individuals' problems in the here and now.

The theorist excludes certain aspects of the group from his perception, thus establishing a somewhat artificial hierarchy around what should be given attention in the group. On the other hand, if he subscribes to an orientation toward exploring both group process and unconscious motives for behavior, he is more able to explain and predict a greater number of phenomena.

A third and final feature of the eclectic theoretical approach is that it is more apt to allow for shifts in goals and in the direction of intervention by the group leader. This feature is closely related to the second discussed above in that an approach which explains numerous phenomena is likely to afford a shift in the leader's goals or interventions. Since an eclectically oriented leader can choose to focus on a broad number of phenomena, he has several options regarding which set of goals and interventions will be employed at any one time. He may, in the first two sessions, assist in examining and modifying dysfunctional communication between members. In the third and fourth sessions he may help examine how members' problems relate to basic insecurities in interpersonal relationships or work more closely with members' feelings of here and now. Finally in the closing sessions he may find it appropriate to help the group examine the various phases of development it went through in order to resolve internal uncertainties regarding intimacy and authority. In essence then, the leader could draw on several theoretical orientations—communication, interpersonal, existential, and group dynamics—that would determine the goals and interventions for the group. These goals and interventions would not be based on a unidimensional theoretical orientation, for example, directed solely at examining unconscious motives for members' behavior, but on an eclectic theoretical orientation to group work.

After considering these features of an eclectic theoretical approach, it can be concluded that such an approach has certain advantages and disadvantages as compared to the more unidimensional approach.

One clear advantage of an eclectic orientation is the freedom it allows the practitioner in selection of interventions and goals. This is both desirable from the practitioner's personal point of view and advantageous for the groups he leads. With an eclectic orientation a leader can make decisions about what approach is appropriate for a certain group, as well as what is appropriate for the group members at this particular time.

An eclectic orientation can also be highly desirable to the group theorist. As was indicated earlier, the freedom to shift one's theoretical orientation increases the theorist's ability to explain and predict a greater number of group phenomena. The group theorist is all too aware of the inability of any one theory to describe what goes on in a group and what causes people to interact as they do. The practitioner becomes aware of this problem when he intervenes, and his interventions turn out to be inappropriate, ill timed, or insensitive to the group as a whole. The theorist experiences this problem when he predicts one thing will happen and it does not. Like the practitioner, if the theorist gives attention to only one aspect of the group, for example, communication patterns or individuals' unconscious motivations, he may prove to be off base in predictions about individuals and the group as a whole. Let us consider, for example, the group theorist who predicts certain outcomes on the basis of his knowledge of communication theory. He makes the assumption that as members are made aware of their dysfunctional communication patterns in the group and the environment is supportive, they will abandon these dysfunctional patterns in favor of sending clear messages. What occurs is that members do abandon these dysfunctional patterns but take them up again several sessions later and again at termination time. Some knowledge of common group tensions and group dynamics would have enabled the theorist to predict not only what conditions would foster members' abandonment of their dysfunctional communication patterns but also what conditions would reactivate these patterns in the group. In the middle phases of the group when members are competing for control or at the end when they are struggling with the problem of whether they want to remain dependent on the group, they may revert to former dysfunctional patterns. The theorist's knowledge of both communication and group process theories would have increased his ability to predict certain outcomes in the group, as well as a greater number of phenomena.

Despite the advantages of an eclectic theoretical orientation, there are certain drawbacks. For instance, an eclectic approach rarely has a clear and determinable framework or basis connecting various views. Thus the practitioner may be guided more by his intuition and less by reason when he decides on certain interventions and goals. He may experience feelings of being in limbo or may at times be indecisive about what to do. If this occurs, he is likely to give the impression of not really knowing what he is doing. This may make the group extremely uneasy with his leadership.

The group theorist, like the group practitioner, is also at a disadvantage if he does not have an overall framework to connect his various concepts and principles. An eclectically oriented theorist may not be able to identify the basic assumptions that hold his ideas together, since he has incorporated them at will without being too concerned about building a logical foundation for his choice. Consequently any predictions made may be criticized from the standpoint that his assumptions are not clearly spelled out in advance. His theories may be accused of being unsophisticated and not soundly based.

Clearly, then, if the group practitioner or group theorist is to reap the benefits of an eclectic theoretical approach and not be hampered by its drawbacks, he must be able to delineate the framework that connects the principles and concepts he has gathered from different theories.

The nurse group leader and an eclectic orientation to group work

The advantages of an eclectic theoretical orientation are especially attractive to the nurse group leader. One reason is that an eclectic orientation is suited to the nurse's professional training and education in most schools of nursing. The beginning practitioner in schools of nursing is likely to be exposed to a broad coverage of several theoretical frameworks as opposed to consideration of only one. This is because most nurse educators in mental health or who have adapted mental health concepts in their presentation of nursing principles have themselves been exposed to a variety of theoretical frameworks. Even at the graduate level in psychiatric–

mental health nursing, students may be exposed initially to one particular theory, but usually they graduate with a more eclectic orientation. It is fitting for nurses to fully capitalize on the nature of their education and therefore to adopt an eclectic approach to group work after they leave their training institutions.

The flexibility and freedom an eclectic approach offers the group practitioner has special meaning for nurses. The rationale for some schools of nursing to expose students to a variety of theories is that it presents an opportunity to select aspects of theories most appropriate to their own level of skill and understanding and best suited to their philosophy of nursing. It is characteristic of theories to require students not only to achieve certain skills and knowledge but also to adopt certain philosophies, which may or may not suit them as individuals. For example, the existential and Gestalt theories are based on the idea that man is responsible for himself; no one else can be responsible for him. To some nurses this premise may be foreign and even unacceptable; yet to become an existential group leader they would need to incorporate this premise in their approach to group members. Likewise a full psychoanalytic orientation would require nurses to be trained extensively in the meaning of symbolic behavior and the interpretation of members' problems in light of unconscious fears and wishes. If the underlying philosophy of a theory is acceptable to nurses, they still need to adapt the theory to their particular level of skill and understanding. Since they must be aware of both sophisticated and more basic theoretical frameworks as their career develops, nurse group leaders will find an eclectic orientation more appropriate.

The rationale behind an eclectic approach for nurse group leaders also relates to the fact that such orientation enables nurses to retain a certain degree of flexibility in their role as group practitioners. Some nurses will shift from one work setting to another, for example, from a home for unwed mothers to a general hospital setting, a community health center, or a mental health clinic. When they change environments they will be exposed to different goals. These goals may dictate or limit the type of group work nurses can do and the theoretical orientation needed. In one setting, for example, an interpersonal or communication orientation would be suitable, whereas in another a psychoanalytic or a Gestalt orientation would be more appropriate. If nurses have initially established an eclectic orientation, they will find that their adjustment to these different settings may be eased.

Along these same lines, some nurse group leaders may want to work with a variety of individuals in a variety of settings, that is, with medical-surgical patients or psychiatric inpatients, but also with staff groups or family groups. In this case one orientation, such as a communication orientation, may not be sufficient. They would also need a sound background in group dynamics theory or interpersonal theory. If they expect to work with a variety of members in many different group settings, they will need to understand and apply more than one theoretical framework; again, an eclectic approach would seem to be more suited to them.

It is interesting to point out that for the same reasons this approach is desirable to both beginning and advanced nursing students. Undergraduate students learning group work for the first time have told me that they did not think it was possible or advisable that they use only one theoretical framework. They claimed that using several theories and gaining an understanding of the uses and values of each gave them a broader approach and allowed them to shift focus when one theory became "nonfunctional" due either to the patient situation or to the skill of the leader. Graduate students, likewise, claim that they want to be allowed to utilize premises from more than one theory as they see relevance to their clients and what interventions are called for at different times.

To summarize, an eclectic theoretical approach to group work has certain advantages and disadvantages. The advantages of such an approach have special meaning for nurse group leaders, given their current preparation in schools of nursing, the need to adapt a theory to their own level of skill and philosophy of nursing, as well as the requirements placed on them in different work settings with different types of groups. The conclusion was drawn that an eclectic orientation seems to be better suited to the nurse than is a unidimensional orientation.

Before ending this chapter, however, it is important to address ourselves to the disadvantages of this approach and how they may be overcome. First, it is my belief that some beginning nurse practitioners may find security in exposure to one theory in depth. I suggest, for example, that the beginning group worker become thoroughly familiar with one of the theories most frequently employed by group practitioners as presented in Chapter 6. Once the student has acquired an understanding of the concepts, principles, and assumptions contained therein, it is appropriate for him to explore other theories. The references cited at the end of Chapter 6 will be helpful in selecting reading material pertinent to the theoretical frameworks discussed here. As the student becomes aware of differences and similarities in these theories, he may find himself being drawn toward one or more sets of concepts and principles. The students who find themselves moving toward an eclectic orientation have the responsibility to determine what underlying premises govern their selection of some principles and concepts and their rejection of others. They will most likely benefit from the guidance and inquiry of their instructors in determining and formulating the basis of their orientation. When this has been accomplished, they not only will reap the benefits offered by an eclectic orientation but also will successfully avoid the drawbacks of such an approach.

REFERENCES

1. Coleman, J., and Broen, W.: Abnormal psychology and modern life, Glenview, Ill., 1972, Scott, Foresman and Co., p. 664.
2. Fromm-Reichmann, F.: Principles of intensive psychotherapy, Chicago, 1950, The University of Chicago Press.
3. Schutz, W.: The ego, FIRO theory and the leader as completer (reprint), New York, 1968, Holt, Rinehart & Winston.
4. Whitaker, D. S., and Liebermann, M. A.: Psychotherapy through the group process, New York, 1964, Atherton Press.
5. Wiener, D.: A practical guide to psychotherapy, New York, 1968, Harper & Row, Publishers.

SUGGESTED READING

Slavson, S. R.: Eclecticism versus sectarianism in group psychotherapy, Int. J. Group Psychother. **20:**3-13, 1970.

DEFINITION EXERCISE FOR PART TWO

As a review of Part Two and as a guide for surveying the literature about each theoretical framework discussed, try defining the following concepts. As you define each concept within each framework, try to determine how one concept fits with another under the same framework and what implications they have for the study and practice of group work.

I. Psychoanalytic concepts
 Unconscious
 Preconscious
 Conscious
 Id
 Ego and group ego
 Superego
 Group mind
 Basic drives or instincts
 Transference
 Countertransference
 Eros
 Thanatos
 Primary process
 Secondary process
 Gratification
 Cathexis
 Libido
II. Interpersonal concepts
 Interpersonal
 Anxiety
 Interpersonal security
 Security operation
 Self-system
 Good me
 Bad me
 Not me
 Good mother
 Bad mother
 Consensual validation
 Parataxic distortion
 Parataxic
 Prototaxic mode
 Syntaxic mode
 Selective inattention
III. Communication concepts
 Nonverbal communication
 Disturbed communication
 Therapeutic
  communication
 Feedback
 Checking-out
 Acknowledgment
 Acknowledgment with
  understanding

Acknowledgment without
 understanding
Negative feedback
Positive feedback
Overload
Underload
Tangential reply or
 tangential response
Communication networks
Denotative level of
 communication
Metacommunicative level
 of communication
Complementary interaction
Symmetrical interaction
Communication syndromes
Disqualification
Spokesmanship
Double-level messages
Congruency and mutual fit
Request value of messages
Model communicator
Dysfunctional
 communicator
Functional communicator
IV. Group dynamics and group
  process concepts
 Group process
 Group dynamics
 Stage or phase of a group
 Common group tensions
 Group goals
 Group culture
 Group focal conflicts
 Group cohesion
 Group themes
 Group equilibrium
 Group norms or standards
 Group leadership
 Consensual validation
 Group problem solving and
  group decision making
 Members' roles or group
  task roles
 Group maintenance
  functions

V. Existential and Gestalt
  concepts
 Gestalt
 Reality
 Freedom
 Self (not me and me)
 Psychological health
 Creativity
 Awareness
 Experience and
  experiencing
 Self-actualization
 Ego-states
 Desensitization
 Transcend
 Projection, introjection, and
  retroflexion
 Contact and contact
  boundary
 Organism environment
  field
 "I-thou" relationship
VI. Behavior modification
  concepts
 Adaptive/maladaptive
  behavior
 Operant behavior
 Reinforcement (positive/
  negative/neutral)
 Extinction of behavior
 Schedules of reinforcement
 Temporal gradient of
  reinforcement
 Operant and respondent
  conditioning
 Satiation/deprivation
 Baseline data
 Reinforcement history
 Discriminative stimulus
 Behavior program:
  prompts; fading shaping;
  successive approxima-
  tions; token systems; star
  charts

119

*

PART THREE

The practice of group work

The outcomes of group work are a direct result of the interaction between membership features, group structural properties, and leadership characteristics. Group leaders are able to influence all three variables. They may decide what constitutes a membership criterion, for example, and match leadership skills with given objectives.

This important and pervasive influence of the leader(s) can be likened to that of the architect whose interest as a social engineer is to facilitate an adequate design so that some basic purposes can be met by the people utilizing the framework.

The leader(s) establishes a "floor" plan for the group, specifying organizational and structural properties that influence the outcome of the group. The "interior," that is, the topics that get discussed, the specific relationships between members, is in large part reflective of the unique individuals that compose the groups and how they choose to deal with problems within the limits set forth.

The presence and skill of the leader(s) will impact on the resolution of problems, change in behavior, and the insight members glean. Unlike the architect, the group leader(s) in a group therapy or group therapeutic group does not hand over the design to a competent contractor and his team of task-oriented workers. Quite the contrary, the leader(s) continues to play an integral role in the determination of the group's outcomes via group maintenance, role modeling, and insight-promoting functions.

As a group maintenance agent the leader(s) fosters group cohesion and recognizes factors that lead to divisiveness in the group, for example, subgrouping, absences, and scapegoating. The leader(s) also reinforces norms and behaviors that are conducive to therapeutic aims, for example, self-disclosure, involvement, and nonjudgmental acceptance. As promoter of the group's (and individual's) insight into areas of group and communication processes, the leader(s) significantly affects the quality of the therapeutic experience and members' ability to take responsibility for thoughts, attitudes, and behavior.

The chapters included in Part Three of the text will elucidate these statements about the practice of group work. An eclectic theoretical framework guides a discussion of basic leadership functions and interventions in a wide variety of group settings in Chapter 8 and the identification of principles in the establishment, maintenance, and termination of a therapeutic or group therapy group in Chapter 9. Practice illustrations are found in these chapters, but to even a greater extent in Chapter 10, which presents various case studies that depict how the leader(s) uses a theoretical framework in analyzing and intervening in practice situations.

Basic leadership functions and interventions

Introduction

In Part One of this text we outlined the numerous groups with which nurses may be involved as group leaders. These groups were categorized as being group therapy, therapeutic, self-actualization, and reference groups. We explained that nurses could be working with various client populations including individuals of all ages in groups established for particular therapeutic purposes or in preexisting groups, for example, the family, work groups, a classroom of students, or a neighborhood youth gang. We indicated that, although some of their clients may have frank overt signs of mental illness, nurses may also work with persons who are merely seeking further self-actualization, who need assistance at a time of physical or emotional crisis, or who want to solve a particular problem or alter a habit. For nurses who decide to lead groups composed of clients with such needs, the question arises: how must they function in order to ensure the benefits of group membership to their clients. It is important to devote some time to discussing what basic leadership functions may be applicable to the role of the nurse group leader or nurse group therapist. These functions having been outlined, various interventions appropriate for the nurse in light of leadership functions in the group will be enumerated. It is important to note that all those interventions useful to nurses or helpful to their clients will not be covered; rather, only those interventions essential to the nurse's role in guiding the group as a whole and in acting as a change agent with reference to individual member's concerns will be mentioned.

The idea of common group leadership functions is not new. Many of the basic group psychotherapy texts either explicitly enumerate or implicitly suggest various functions that need to be fulfilled by the leader or group therapist. Some of these texts are Kadis's *A Practicum of Group Psychotherapy,*[6] Johnson's *Group Therapy — A Practical Approach,*[5] and Yalom's *The Theory and Practice of Group Psychotherapy.*[11] In addition Marilyn Schurman[10] enumerates five functions she views as especially appropriate for the nurse group therapist. Basically they include (1) orienting individuals to the group, (2) helping members check out their thoughts and feelings, (3) redirecting questions so that they are answered by members, (4) helping all members to participate, and (5) acting as a resource person.

Quite often what these authors describe as leadership functions are, more appropriately, specific leadership interventions. In this discussion of functions and interventions I attempt to make clear the differences between the two—a function on the one hand and an intervention on the other hand. A function here is more precisely the purpose of the leader in the group. An intervention, as opposed to a function, is the specific act or set of activities that nurses employ to accomplish their purpose in the group. For example, the nurse may encourage members to share common problems. This intervention refers to activities that are appropriate with reference to the nurse's function—facilitating the benefits of group membership. The rationale behind interventions provides the logical link between the nurse's purpose in the group and the nurse's actual behavior. Using this same example, the nurse might encourage members to share common problems in the group in order to reduce members' feelings of isolation. If feelings of isolation are minimized, members may realize the security of belonging to a group, one benefit of group membership.

Differentiating between group leadership functions and leadership interventions allows me to talk about the possibility that any one individual in the group may effect an intervention that is directly related to the function or purpose of the group leader. But leadership functioning is typically the domain or purpose for a group leader and not why members have joined the group. This differentiation is extremely important when leaders are tempted to relinquish their leadership role or depend on members to act as a "coleader" or "cotherapist." Even in self-growth groups, for example, a sensitivity group where it is appropriate to encourage members to assume the leadership role, the leader should be aware that his purpose in the group is to function as a leader; members are not responsible for intervening as a leader at all times. In addition it is sometimes the case that a group therapist will shift the role of leader in the group in order to prompt a patient to perform some leadership function in the group; he employs a sound rationale; for example, it will increase this patient's self-esteem as well as mobilize the other patients more quickly. The therapist who experiments with these techniques in the group must be aware of the fact that he is not allowing this member to seek the same type of assistance others are offered and that he may isolate this member from the group as a whole. The differentiation here between leadership function and leadership interventions hopefully clarifies to a greater extent why a member may take on leadership interventions but why leadership functions are more the domain of the group leader.

Leadership functions

Leadership is basic to effective group experience.[1] It contributes to the attainment of group goals, the viability of the group for members, and effective interaction—in short, to group performance. This discussion describes four basic leadership functions appropriate for nurse group leaders. These functions pertain to their role regardless of what type of group they lead and regardless of the client composition of their group. They are general and global but give the reader a good indication of what the role of the nurse group leader can be.

First the group leader facilitates benefits of group membership. Certain natural benefits have been ascribed to all groups. Groups are believed to meet people's needs for security, for belonging, and for companionship. They are thought to provide members an opportunity for realization of individual capacities, as well as opportunities to develop a type of community consciousness.[9]

The group leader, by establishing a group, starts a process by which members can meet their needs for security, belonging, and companionship. In addition he can take several steps that might enhance the fulfillment of these needs in the group once the group has begun. Leaders can, for example, increase the interdependence of members on one another, foster members' sharing of common interests, and outline a direction for the group. For example, in the first meeting of an outpatient group the leader suggested that each member tell the group something about the problems that brought them to the clinic, prefacing the request with the explanation that they do have something in common because they have the same emotional disorder. Each member responded by telling the group his problem. This activity stimulated members to ask one another about shared symptoms and minimized some beginning concerns of being together with people you do not know.

Such interventions will help to increase members' feelings of security, belongingness, and companionship in the group. It is important that leaders know how to facilitate the achievement of these natural benefits of group membership, especially if the structure of the group is such that it does not easily afford full benefits to its members. In short-term groups it is very important that leaders know how to stimulate (or simulate) situations that will encourage feelings of belongingness and security. It is thought that a group needs time to develop a sense of belongingness and cohesion, time which is not available to many short-term, abbreviated group experiences.

Second the group leader maintains a viable group atmosphere. As was indicated above, nurses are in a position to safeguard and enhance the natural benefits of group membership. Closely related to this function is the ability to maintain a viable group atmosphere in which persons are free to be present, free to talk about what concerns them, and free to experiment with new behaviors without severe threat. It is not unusual for nurses to let the group escape undue tension, for example, by avoiding the subject, if this helps to keep the group intact and to increase members' safety in the group. In some ways their function to maintain a viable group atmosphere parallels what Cartwright and Zander[1] describe as "group maintenance" functions: to keep interpersonal relations pleasant, or if not pleasant, relatively safe. Without the leader's attempt to ensure a viable atmosphere minus undue stress and anxiety, there is always the possibility that the group will not learn from one another and will not be able to remain intact.

An example of how important this factor is can be illustrated by a group therapy experience where the leaders were relatively passive to the verbal abuse one member was giving another. Instead of interrupting the accusatory, angry verbal whipping one male patient was giving another, the therapists let it go on until one member left the group and another said she would not come back. Before the group arrived at disbanding as a solution to communication difficulties the leaders could have intervened to redirect the quality of interaction and make it safe for all members to remain. Although the group can be reassembled, not all members will be willing to come, and there is little the leaders can do to insist on it, since they demonstrated previously that they could not keep the group intact.

A third function of the group leader is to oversee group growth. According to Cartwright and Zander,[1] most groups have goals. In less formalized groups these goals might not be explicit; still there is some defined reason that keeps members together and that guides the growth of the group. In groups such as group therapy, therapeutic, and self-growth groups, the goals may be specific and explicit. A self-help group, for example, may have the goal of encouraging members to alter a habit, for example, smoking. This is a therapeutic goal with which all members identify if they join the group. A self-actualization group may have the goal of increasing one's awareness of how members interact with one another in the group. Whatever the goal of the group, the leaders have a direct responsibility to the achievement of this goal and to the group's progress in meeting it. They have the responsibility to ascertain the growth or movement of the group toward its goals.

In his role as observer of group growth the leader may keep members' attention on the goals, clarify issues in terms of how they relate to the goals, and evaluate the group's progress toward the goals periodically and with the assistance of members. In some task-oriented groups the secretary who is recording group decisions is the person who is delegated the responsibility of summarizing group attitudes and asking for clarification about where the group stands on an issue.

Reminding the group of its purposes and denoting progress serves to redirect group efforts as pointed out in this sensitivity group experience. The group leader relinquished active participation and aroused anxiety in members who began to lose track of why they were meeting. In an attempt to relieve their anxiety, members demanded the leader tell them what they should talk about. Realizing the leader would not oblige them specifically, but merely said, "You are here to learn about group process," they decided that perhaps they were learning and did not know it. The group, with the assistance of the leader, began then to examine what was happening and what this had to do with group process.

Fourth and finally the group leader regulates individual member's growth within the group setting. Individual members frequently proceed toward meeting group objectives at different rates; in addition the leader may formulate specific and more particularized objectives for some members' experience in the group. For these reasons he will be concerned with regulating individual member's growth in the group as well as with enhancing total group movement toward group goals. One objective of a married couples group would be to decrease the couples' use of dysfunctional communication patterns with one another and in the group. For one spouse to meet this objective, he must first be able to perceive that he was communicating in a dysfunctional manner. His partner and the rest of the couples may be aware that they communicate dysfunctionally and are ready to explore why or what alternatives they have in communicating to one another. Still the leaders would need to facilitate this one member's awareness of how he communicates before he would be at the same level of readiness to experiment as the others in the group. When the leader intervenes with respect to one member, he is concerned not only with the progress of the total group but also with concentrating on individuals' growth within the group.

At any one stage his interventions may be more individualized than global, and therefore not solely directed toward the general maintenance and success of the group.

Leadership interventions

Many behaviors may have significance with respect to the four group leadership functions outlined above. Not all of these actions may come from the group leaders per se. Group needs, for example, for goal achievement and group maintenance may be fulfilled simultaneously by one or more members or by the actions of the designated leaders and members.[1] The interventions discussed here are typical leadership actions or activities. They are appropriate for the nurse in any group setting and are designed to help fulfill leadership functions in the group, that is, to facilitate benefits of group membership, to maintain a viable group atmosphere, to oversee group growth, and to regulate individual members' growth within the group.

Outlining and interpreting group objectives

In the beginning sessions of the group, as well as throughout the life of the group, the leader can outline and interpret the objectives he holds for the group and its members. In group therapy groups this activity is referred to as establishing a group "contract." The leader specifies for the group his objectives, and in the case where members themselves are devising goals for the group, he helps the group clarify these goals. Usually when goals are being specified, a more general plan of how goals will be met, including how long the group will meet, the ground rules, and so on, is also specified.

It is very important from the standpoint of fostering a viable group atmosphere that members have an understanding of what is expected of them. A group that operates without any clearly defined goals can arouse undue anxiety in its members. Although coming into a new group is something members may have done many times, it is not without the tension associated with unknown aspects of a new experience. The leader can minimize the anxiety felt by members in the group by working to clarify the direction the group should be taking and how the group might progress toward meeting group objectives. For example, the leader might explain to one group that the goal is for members to share with one another the perceptual problems they have that were caused by their recent eye surgery. In addition the leader might suggest that the group begin by everyone's explaining what it was like after his surgery. If the group was a sensitivity group instead of a therapeutic group of eye patients, the leader might explain that the purpose of the group is for members to learn how they are perceived by others in the group. Likewise the leader might suggest that one mode of proceeding in this direction would be to start by going around the group and telling persons your first impressions of them.

It is a vital need of the group to know where it is expected to go and how it might get there. Outlining and interpreting group objectives can serve to meet this need and decrease members' anxieties about the unknown aspects of the group experience. The leader's role here cannot be overemphasized.

Manipulating physical and structural arrangements

In establishing groups the leader may have at his disposal several decisions that can enhance the participation of members and make for the success of the group. These decisions concern structural and physical arrangements of the groups, for example, how many members in the group, whether the group should be open to new members or essentially closed to newcomers, how frequently and for what duration the group should meet, and the specific locale of the group, including seating arrangements and so on. Sometimes decisions such as these are dictated by the agencies in which the nurse is operating. That is, the type of client, the number of clients, and the physical surroundings may be predetermined to some extent for the nurse. In this case the leader must be aware of how these predetermined conditions may affect the groups, but he has fewer decisions to make about the structural and physical arrangements of his group. Whereas a more extensive discussion of these leadership decisions is taken up in Chapter 9, dealing with the assemblage of a group therapy group, I have chosen to outline basic considerations here as well.

Although the composition and duration of the group depend on many things, for example, the goals of the groups and the type of client problems being confronted, other group leaders and I generally suggest the following guidelines. The leader should take care that the composition of his group does not vary to the extent that one or more members could be considered isolates or "different." That is, if members do vary in age, intelligence, education, race, marital status, severity of their emotional problems, or any other important personal feature, this variance should not be so great as to lead to separation and isolation of any member in the group. It is usually a good idea that members do, however, vary in the extent to which they are talkative or silent, ascendant or submissive.

The size of the groups can vary, too, depending on the purpose of the groups and the goals of the leader for the group. Usually a group of about eight to twelve members is advisable. Yalom and Terrazas[12] suggest that groups become less effective if they contain fewer than four or five active members. Likewise Coffey[2] warns that any number over twenty is more of an assemblage and probably does not offer the benefits that smaller groups can.

The issue of whether to have an "open" or "closed" group again depends on the purpose and objectives for the group. It is unlikely that a leader would choose a format where members could be added during the process of the group once the group has begun, however. Continually adding new members has the effect of disrupting ongoing interaction and inhibiting cohesion in the group. Still an "open" format, as opposed to a "closed" group, does have the advantage of offering more coverage to a greater number of clients, especially when turnover of members in the group is great. In the future, as nurses move into new areas of group work in the community at large, they may have little control over whether their groups are captive, cohesive groups or constantly changing aggregates of individuals. It is important that they know how to operate effectively under both conditions—open and closed formats.

The duration and length of sessions is likewise a decision based on the goals of the group and the nature of members' concerns. Some groups, for example, those for the purpose of altering a habit, may extend indefinitely and be available to members two or more hours daily. Other groups such as marathon encounter groups may extend over an abbreviated period, perhaps for 24 hours, but demand a concentrated effort on the part of the group. It is frequently the case with other than special problem groups and marathon groups that the average duration of the group may be one to several months, for 60 to 90 minutes biweekly or weekly. The length of each session is far more common, however, than the duration of the group. This is because leaders seem to have formulated more definite opinions about what can be done in one session and how long different clients can tolerate and benefit by a single session. Frequently the decision about the duration of the group experience is predetermined by the doctor's evaluation of the patients' needs, by the length of the term—if the group is offered as a course, or by the overall length of hospitalization if the group is an adjunct to members' treatment in an inpatient general hospital or mental health center.

The physical and environmental conditions in which the group is to operate have received much attention but cannot be overstressed. A leader who chooses to run marathon groups cannot deny the impact that ventilation, seating arrangements, and lighting can have on the group. A leader who chooses to run group psychotherapy groups with acutely ill psychotic patients cannot overlook the spacing of members in the room and whether there are noises or movement outside the room that will easily distract members. Although there is little substantial data to support this, leaders do feel that certain physical arrangements can affect the moods of members, as well as their degree of sociability and their trust in the group. Leaders should do their best to alter the environment so that it elicits emotional comfort and provides a sense of boundary but does not pin members in and is not at odds with their objectives for the group. Increasing members' awareness of their feelings toward one another, for example, can be hampered by a closed, stale room where members are lulled into an apathetic state by the humdrum noise of traffic outside the window.

Increasing interaction between members

To facilitate the benefits of group membership the leader must stimulate verbal interaction between members in the group. It is through this type of interaction that members get an idea about how they fit with each other and how they fit in the group, and thus develop some sense of belongingness, security, and companionship. It is also through this interaction that members begin to share common problems and learn from each other.

It is not always easy, however, to stimulate verbal exchange that would be both helpful and rewarding for individuals in the group. Communication theorists come to our aid here by suggesting that individuals do have a basic need and desire to communicate and to be understood—that the process of communicating itself is rewarding.[8] Individuals like to communicate and to be understood; therefore any interaction that can lead to verbal exchange and mutual understanding in the group is likely to be rewarding, especially for the participants.

The leader can employ several techniques to stimulate interaction. Basic inter-

Table 1. Interviewing skills

Interviewing technique by the leader(s)	Group member response	Outcome
1. *Giving information:* "My purpose in offering this group experience is . . ."	*Further validate* his assumptions: "How is this going to happen?"	Leader(s) and member(s) enter into a dialogue in which member(s) get more information to make decisions and build trust in group experience.
2. *Seeking clarification:* "Did you say you were upset with John because he said that?"	*May try to restate* his thoughts or feelings: "Yes, I guess I was upset?"	Member becomes aware that he was not clear and learns to identify thoughts and feelings more precisely, at the same time taking responsibility for them.
3. *Encouraging description and exploring* (delving further into communication or experiences): "How did you feel when Joann said that to you?"	*Elaborates* on his message: "I didn't like it very much."	Member(s) deal in greater depth with an experience in the group; again taking responsibility for their reactions. (This example also places events in time or sequence—lending further perspective to group events.)
4. *Presenting reality:* "Would other members think Joann was unstable if they interviewed her for a job? You don't appear shaky to me."	*Listens and considers* other possibilities.	Member compares perception of self with others' perception of him.
5. *Seeking consensual validation* (seek mutual understanding of what is being communicated): "Did I understand you to say that you feel better now than you did last week?"	*Further clarification:* "Well, yes, I'm better than last week but not as good as I'd like to be."	Group and leader(s) learn how member views his progress and in what way they should receive his evaluation of himself.
6. *Focusing* (identifying a single topic to concentrate on): "Maybe we could identify one problem you have and talk more about that."	*Channels thinking:* Members may think of the most puzzling problem they have.	Group and leader(s) identify specific topics they can resolve before the meeting ends. They increase their understanding of one problem before jumping to others.
7. *Encouraging comparison* (asking members to compare and contrast their experiences with others in the group): "How did the rest of the group handle this problem?"	*Group members share* their experiences as they relate to the topic.	Leader(s) and members gain greater insight into their commonalities and differences and learn from one another alternative ways of responding to problems.

Table 1. Interviewing skills—cont'd

Interviewing technique by the leader(s)	Group member response	Outcome
8. *Making observations:* "You look more comfortable now, John, than you did at the beginning of the meeting."	*Group members have something to respond to:* "I feel more at ease now."	Group members and leader(s) place attention on significant events and can elaborate on their meaning.
or	or	
"The group has been silent for the last 5 minutes."	"I think we are quiet because we are bored."	
9. *Giving recognition or acknowledging:* "John, you are new to the group. Perhaps we can introduce ourselves."	*Feels acknowledged and included:* "Yes, I'm John and I came here because . . ."	Members view specific instances as important, and the leader(s) reinforce the behavior or event they choose to notice; in this case, the desire to come to group.
10. *Accepting* (not necessarily agreeing with but receiving communication with openness): "Yes, I hear you say that you don't know if you want to be in the group or not."	*Feels heard and understood* without fear of attack.	Members learn that even "nonacceptable" attitudes can be talked about, and perhaps any thought is not so horrible that they cannot share it.
11. *Encouraging evaluation* (asking the group as a whole or individual members to judge their experience): "When Marilyn gives you support do you feel better?"	*Members reflect* on progress made: "Not exactly, because I don't know if I can trust her to be honest."	The criteria for success becomes clearer to members, and new directions may be formulated as a result of the discussion.
or	or	
"How did we do in helping Joann with her problem?"	"It was hard. I'd like to know from her."	
12. *Summarizing* (encapsulating in a few sentences what has occurred): "The group discussed several issues and problems today—they were . . ."	*Members recall* significant points and close off consideration of new or extraneous topics.	Members and leader(s) place events in perspective, identifying salient points of a group session. Such a summary can lead to a better understanding of group process.

viewing and communication skills are most helpful. He can offer leading statements or merely ask direct or indirect questions. For example: "Go on George and tell me what you are experiencing," is a leading statement, which incidentally is a mild command to encourage verbal participation. "What are you thinking?" directed to the group as a whole is an open-ended question and identifies no particular person in the group—leaving it open as to who answers and what is discussed. "What do you feel about that, Sara?" is a direct question that leaves no doubt about who should respond.

There are many basic interviewing techniques useful for stimulating verbal interaction in a group, both among members and between the leader and different members. The reader is encouraged to brush up on some of the basic interviewing techniques outlined by Hilegard Peplau in her "Interpersonal Techniques: The Crux of Psychiatric Nursing,"[7] by Garrett in *Interviewing: Its Principles and Methods*,[3] and by Hayes and Larson in *Interacting With Patients*.[4]

Table 1 is a synopsis of some important interviewing skills that I have found to be extremely useful as a group leader. An example of how these strategies are used, the possible response of group member(s), and expected outcomes are illustrated.

In addition to the many verbal promptings the leader can utilize to stimulate interaction, there are other modes of increasing interaction. The leader can use audio and visual aids, recreation, games, or commonplace situations such as eating a meal together to stimulate verbal interaction between members. Modes of increasing interaction between members in groups have taken on many creative and interesting forms from a hairdressing session to group problem-solving tasks. The reader should keep in mind that these techniques are not ends in themselves, but means to an end. With increased verbal interaction in the group, members are more likely to share common concerns and benefit from group membership.

Encouraging the sharing of common problems

Closely related to the activity of increasing verbal interaction in the group is the intervention of encouraging the sharing of common problems. The purpose of increasing interaction is quite frequently to get members to share their common concerns and learn from each other. Group meetings seem to assume a greater meaning and interest when members focus on issues relevant to all or most of the group.[11] But also, if members share their common interests, concerns, and problems, they are more likely to form bonds of commonality with others. A group that has established areas of commonality confers a sense of acceptance and support to its members.

The leader should be alert to common issues or problems in the group and reinforce these subjects for the group to deal with. These may involve shared experiences in the group or outside the group or feelings such as loneliness, fear, or discouragement. In the beginning of the group, what members learn about each other that they have in common may be superficial and tangential to what the group is supposed to discuss. The leader should not block these discussions because their purpose is extremely important; that is, they establish bonds between individuals in the group that make it easier for members to deal next with more important areas and more emotionally ladened concerns. Members, by "feeling each other out" in reference to what seem to be the most mundane topics, for example, "Where do you live? Oh, I live two miles from there;" or "Did you like those beans we had for lunch? I didn't," get a better indication of how they are like and unlike others in the group and who is likely to support them in the future. In essence this type of dialogue is members' attempt to establish their own security in the group. Once they feel more comfortable in the group, the leader can and should expect them to stick more closely to what the group is expected to discuss. It is wise to encourage the group to proceed at its own pace from sharing what seem to be irrelevant aspects of their lives to more significant experiences.

Groups that fail to formulate areas of commonality suffer problems of fragmentation and also induce anxiety in members. This problem is noted in Chapter 10 with reference to case study 2—"Individual inclusion and group cohesion problems in multiple family group therapy." Members in this group experienced a gap between themselves and others. This had the effect of causing undue anxiety in certain members and of making it difficult for some members to remain in the group.

Employing strategies with individuals

There may be many instances in a group when the nurse will decide that some strategy is necessary in order to, for example, increase interaction between members or encourage members to discover underdeveloped areas of the self. These strategies are often referred to as techniques and are directed at the group as a whole or at individuals within the group. Tactics like these are taken up in detail in Part Four of this text. The strategy we will concern ourselves with here is that which can be employed to discourage self-injurious behavior in the group.

Certain behaviors on the part of a member can present problems to the group but also impair the individual's ability to relate to others in a group setting. These behaviors can block group growth, as well as inhibit the individual's adaptation of an acceptable role in the group. What could be a generally viable group atmosphere becomes frustrating for some members and destructive for the person exhibiting the destructive behavior. The leader has the otpion of analyzing such behavior in terms of total group process, but most likely will need at some point to intervene to alter the particular member's way of behaving. The behaviors we will take up here are (1) monopolizing, (2) bizarre thinking and acting, and (3) uninvolvement.

Monopolizing behavior on the part of one or more members in the group can have the effect of preventing others in the group from profiting from the group experience. Members tend to resent the monopolizer but may not always be able to deal with him successfully. If they try to stop the monopolizer by indicating their anger at him, they are likely to make him more anxious and therefore provoke him to relieve his anxiety by additional verbalization.

One seemingly successful tactic I have employed and which is talked about by Yalom and Terrazas[12] is to handle the problem initially as a group problem. That is, to consider that when monopolizing behavior occurs, it is encouraged or allowed by others in the group. The leader may suggest that the group look at why one person in the group was given the sole responsibility of the meeting or for the discussion. With this tactic the leader often stimulates the emergence of reasons why members feel uncomfortable in the group: "I don't know anybody here," or "I don't know what to talk about so I let Phil talk." In turn the monopolizer may voice his position, for example, that he really did not know what to talk about either, but "I can't stand silence." With these openings the leader and the group have a much better understanding of what the group needs and how these needs are manifested in the current concerns of members. The leader can help members put their experience in perspective by suggesting that feelings of not knowing what to talk about are normal in the beginning of the group. He can focus on how the group can solve these problems together. He can also relate to the group how, because of discomforts, members assign each other responsibility for the group when these members may not want the burdens bestowed on them.

It is not always the case that someone who monopolizes will respond to this intervention and stop monopolizing. Likewise the group itself may still let one or two members carry the ball for the rest of the group. If this is the case, then the leader may have to come in very firmly and stop the monopolizing behavior. He can employ various methods of intervening: "Now, Ed, wait just a minute," merely stops the monopolizer for a moment. "Stop talking, Ed, I want to hear what Edith and Joe think about this," not only stops the monopolizer but also redirects the discussion to others in the group. The effect of this active interruption on the part of the leader is helpful to the group and the monopolizer. It is a message to the monopolizer that the leader sees and understands the bind he is in, and it communicates to the group that he plans to redirect a frustrating experience that has developed as a result of group impotence.

It is not unusual that excessive monopolizing behavior in a group, especially in a group of acutely ill patients, is a sign of severe anxiety and cannot be handled in the group. In such a situation it is no longer beneficial for the member to remain in the group. The leader may decide to allow the member to move around in the group, to move in and out of the room, or simply to be absent until his anxiety has been abated with medication. Anxiety is the root of the problem, and although a strong leader can do much to increase the security of the member in the group, he must acknowledge the realistic limitations of his role in the group to allay individual member's fears.

Members with bizarre thinking and behavior, especially those experiencing delusions, hallucinations, or other forms of frightening behaviors, present a dificult problem to the group. It is important for the leader to remember the basis of this behavior when he employs certain tactics in the group. Delusions and hallucinations consist of relatively fixed false beliefs that cannot be eliminated with the use of rational argumentation. As soon as a leader attempts to discourage an individual's presentation of fixed beliefs, the member is likely to respond as if this were a severe threat and defensively argue in favor of his ideas. His irrational response will, in turn, accentuate his bizarreness in the group.

I, as well as other leaders of groups with chronic and acute psychiatric patients, believe that far more headway can be made if the leader attempts to pick up on aspects of the member's communication that can be understood and that may be shared by others in the group.

One bizarre member in a group I was leading stated that " . . . the people in this place, they railroaded me here; that's because they knew I had some information that would expose them. They can't risk my getting facts about this place to the President." Instead of confronting this member with the falseness of his belief, I remarked, "You seem to have ideas about the hospital staff and how you got here, Rob; in fact, probably everybody here has certain ideas about why they are here and how they might be helped. Let's hear from others in the group what they hope to gain by being here." This tactic had some disadvantages but also accomplished some ends with the bizarre patient. By this strategy I acknowledged that part of the bizarre member's communication could be understood and shared by others. It prevented him from being totally isolated from others by reinforcing his ability to contribute to the group. The more the leader would have allowed this member to appear "strange," "crazy," or "different" in the group, the more likely the group would exclude any contribution from this member. Exclusion and isolation of the bizarre member may increase his anxiety and intensify his maladaptive or self-impairing behavior. He is acutely aware of being ignored and considered despicable, reactions that confirm for him his deepest concern that he is totally unworthy, useless, and "ugly"—not worth the attention and consideration a "normal" human being would elicit.

A second example of bizarre or isolative behavior that a group leader could confront is that which appears different because it does not fit the context of the group discussion. Tangential or irrelevant talking can occur in any group, and it is important to know how to deal with it.

One member of a medication clinic group brought up what appeared to be a meaningless story in the middle of a discussion of how patients can be helped. He wanted to relate stories about his work and to illustrate the stories with jokes. Surprised at the irrelevancy of his tangent, one leader let him go on, puzzling about how the group would get back on the subject. Finally, waiting to the end of one joke, the leaders actively intervened, replying that his point was well taken—seeing how it partially fit—and then redirecting the conversation to members who had been previously cut off.

Uninvolvement is a common problem in many groups. Members may indicate their uninvolvement by being preoccupied with other things, such as a book, by missing sessions regularly, by sleeping during a meeting, or by simply not participating in discussions of any kind. Sometimes this uninvolvement means disinterest; still it can also indicate anxiety, fear, or hostility on the part of the uninvolved member. It is usually received with much frustration and discouragement by the leader and other members who want the group to succeed and who implicitly evaluate success in terms of "everyone's participating."

The leader must decipher the meaning of the member's uninvolvement. If this uninvolvement relates to the fact that the member is fearful of getting close to others in the group and of exposing himself, then the leader will do well not to force this member to participate too much, too fast. Individuals should be allowed to proceed toward closeness at their own rate, that rate which is comfortable for them. It is often the case that once the group becomes more cohesive, the uninvolved member will feel safe in getting involved and will increase his active participation in the group. It is important that others in the group understand that fear and distrust of the group may motivate individuals to remain aloof. These feelings are far more acceptable and understandable to the group than apparent disinterest, haughtiness, or detachment.

Allowing members to proceed at their own rate in getting involved does not mean that the leader should completely ignore the apparent uninvolvement. On the contrary the nurse should encourage the uninvolved members to participate more actively. If this is the case in a task-oriented group and the nurse leader has discouraged involvement because of leader dominance, then it is important to ease up and let others contribute to the subject and direction of the topic. Members cannot readily experience a sense of belonging in the group unless they do enter in more actively by being present at group sessions, attending to what is going on, and participating in the discussions. If a member is aware that the leader is behind him, attempting at different times to bring him into the group and yet is not pushing him faster than he can go, he is likely to feel supported and is more likely to risk further involvement. For example, members missing sessions or refusing to come have been encouraged by the leader to come and listen. Once they are in the group, if they seem distracted, unattentive, or apathetic, the leader can enlist them directly, for example, to give their opinions about an issue or to relate their experiences. If the member is able to express himself in the group, I acknowledge his ability and reinforce the fact that his opinions, like those of other members, are helpful to the group as a whole. Leaders must be aware, however, that although they are helping an uninvolved member to invest more in the group, they may also be singling this member out to receive special gratification from the leader. Initially this approach may be both useful and necessary, but as the uninvolved member participates more and more in the group, leaders must be on guard that they do not make him overly dependent on their assistance and do not continue the special status they have given him in the group. If they do, they not only may limit this member's capacity for independent growth but also may continue to set him apart from the rest of the group, thereby perpetuating the isolation that they hoped to prevent in the first place.

Reducing undue anxiety

For members to learn from their group experience and also remain in the group and reap the benefits of group membership, they must be relatively free from excessive anxiety. The sources of anxiety for members in groups are numerous. (The reader is encouraged to review the description of Whitaker and Liebermann's group and nuclear focal benefits given in Chapter 6.) Often they arise from simply being in the group and responding to pressures of becoming involved and intimate with others. Members may fear excessive involvement or exposure because it could result in their being rejected or "found out" by the group. They could be severely censored by members or the leader. These concerns are quite common and not always based on reality; that is, although members may fear censorship and rejection by the group, such reactions may not be likely on the part of others in the group. In addition to these more common and shared concerns of members, each individual member may bring to the group his own specific concerns about how he might be received and treated by the leader, as well as by his peers. Often members are fearful of the "power" they think the leader can use over them—his ability to read their minds and his ability to mobilize the group against or in favor of them. Members may attribute to the leader or to other members characteristics that are not realistically based but that nevertheless cause them to be anxious and fearful in the group.

The anxiety members experience at the beginning of the group can be most troublesome to the leader from the standpoint that the anxiety of members is high, and this is a time when the leader himself is acutely sensitive to the need for eliciting members' commitment to the group, something for them that produces more discomfort than no group experience at all. This issue of beginning anxiety is taken up in detail in Chapter. 9. Under these conditions, maintaining a viable group atmosphere devoid of excessive anxiety is quite often the only task the leader can and should attend to at the time. The initial anxiety of being in the group can be alleviated somewhat if the leader clearly states the purpose of the group and how the group might go about meeting its objectives. His demeanor should be supportive and relatively unobtrusive. It is also helpful if the leader can acknowledge members' discomfort and suggest that this uneasiness will decrease as members get to know one another and the leader himself.

Many of the unknown aspects of a group experience cannot be made known until members interact with each other and develop a history of transactions in the group. The outcome of these experiences themselves can allay members' fears and anxieties about their participation—whether they will be overexposed, whether they will lose control, or whether they will be reprimanded or punished by the leader and others. Members should be encouraged to check out their safety in the group and not be limited by their preconceptions about how they will behave and how others will respond to them. The leader can do much to foster a nonthreatening atmosphere simply by continuing to be supportive, understanding, and nonpunitive toward members. In addition the leader can help members identify their fears about being in the group; once these fears are identified, members can work with them as total group problems, supporting each other in a constructive way. (Hilegard Peplau[7] outlines specific steps that are effective in reducing individual's anxiety; these steps could be adapted for use in a group setting.)

Superimposing a theoretical framework

How a leader will oversee group growth and how he will regulate individual members' growth in the group will depend to a great extent on the particular theories he uses as his frame of reference. His choice of a theoretical framework will determine whether he will focus on the development of problem-solving skills, successful interpersonal relationships, knowledge of group process and group dynamics, altered communication patterns, relief from intrapsychic tensions, restoration of basic social skills, increased self-actualization, or a combination of these. His goals for the group and for individual members, as well as how he perceives what is going on in the group, can be strongly influenced by the particular theoretical framework he superimposes on the group.

If the leader is especially sound in communication theory, for example, he may commit himself to enhancing members' communicative skills and diminishing their use of dysfunctional communication patterns. He will view the progress of the group in terms of how they foster individuals' abilities to relinquish unsatisfactory communication patterns and will view individuals' growth in terms of the progress they make in becoming functional communicators. He will direct many of his interventions to enhance these objectives for the group and the individuals in particular. He may develop an array of techniques and interviewing skills based on his orientation toward communication principles and concepts.

When nurses superimpose a theoretical framework on their role in the group, they further delineate those actions they should take. In this sense they further specify their role in the group and lessen the anxiety they and others have about what their role will be. At the same time they initiate a process of selective inattention whereby the leader and the group preoccupy themselves with some aspects of the group and ignore others. Whenever the leader superimposes a theoretical framework on his study and practice of group work, he needs to be aware of the necessary consequences—to be aware of how what he chooses to openly ignore in the group may affect the group's progress toward its more specific goals. The problems of superimposing a theory are discussed more fully in Chapters 6 and 7.

Superimposing a theoretical framework on the nurses' role in the group is not discouraged here. On the contrary it affords nurses sound rationale to support their interventions and to guide their perceptions of the group. On the other hand, it is important that they realize consequences of superimposing one or more theories on their study and practice of group work.

Summarizing the group's progress toward its goals

Part of the leader's role in monitoring the growth of the group and in facilitating benefits of group membership relates to his activity of summarizing the progress of the group toward its goals. Evaluating group performance is not exclusively reserved for final sessions but is something the leader should be concerned with at the end of each session and continually throughout the life of the group. The group should be able to rely on its leader to keep them on the track toward successful accomplishment of their goals. As an observer—not a member—the leader is in a key position to oversee group growth and continually measure the group's progress toward its goals. The leader, more than anyone else in the group, is the "gatekeeper" of the group's goals. He takes an active part in formulating goals and plays a crucial role in terms of the group's success in meeting its goals. When he monitors the group's movement toward its goals, he is summarizing—if not to the group—at least to himself, the group's progress to date.

It is vitally important that as an objective participant in the group he summarize this progress in terms of what the realistic goals of the group are. It is extremely easy for members, especially if they have had little formal group experience or have entered the group with unrealistic expectations of their experience, to become disappointed with the group and its progress. In turn their disappointment may influence whether they attend additional groups and whether they remain with their current group. If the leader sufficiently clarifies the goals of the group at the outset and points out to members what they can expect, there is less chance of members' holding on to unrealistic and inappropriate expectations. Yet it has been my experience that no matter how clear the goals seem to be at the outset, there is the continual need to redefine, reinterpret, and reinforce these goals throughout the group experience. I maintain that interpreting members' behavior and current group events in terms of movement toward or away from group goals is extremely helpful to members and provides a sense of continuity and perspective that members need when they evaluate their experience in the group.

The leader should be aware that disappointment about the progress of the group expressed by members at the beginning and end of the group may camouflage other feelings members may be experiencing and that he should not always deal with disappointment about the group on face value. For example, if members are threatened in the beginning of the group by the involvement the group requires of them, they may attempt to escape this discomfort by explaining that the group experience is not or could not possibly be of any help to them. This claim can give members the excuse they need to terminate their experience before it begins and before the group has had a chance to prove itself worthy. The leader would be making a mistake only to focus on the success or failure of the group; he must also locate members' needs to avoid the group experience at that point in time.

Conclusion

It is helpful here to briefly summarize this chapter about the functions and interventions of the nurse group leaders. First we presented four basic functions that nurses fulfill as group leaders or group therapists in any group. These are global functions that highlight what the role of the nurse can be in any type of group, with any combination of member problems. Second we enumerated several basic leadership interventions. These are selected interventions and do not exhaust all function-linked interventions available to the nurse group leader. In Chapter 9, instead of focusing on general functions and activities basic to nurse leadership in many kinds of groups, the discussion is more focused on the activities appropriate to leaders of group therapy and group therapeutic groups. Also the focus changes from one of general leadership considerations to group-phase-bound interventions, making the role of the leader even more concrete in the mind of the reader.

REFERENCES

1. Cartwright, D., and Zander, A., editors: Group dynamics—research and theory, ed. 3, New York, 1968, Harper & Row, Publishers, pp. 304, 306, 307.

2. Coffey, H. S.: Group psychotherapy. In Berg, I. A., and Pennington, L. A.: Introduction to clinical psychology, New York, 1966, The Ronald Press Co.
3. Garrett, A.: Interviewing: its principles and methods, New York, 1961, G. P. Putnam's Sons.
4. Hayes, J., and Larson, K.: Interacting with patients, New York, 1963, The Macmillan Co.
5. Johnson, J. A.: Group therapy—a practical approach, New York, 1963, McGraw-Hill Book Co.
6. Kadis, A.: A practicum of group psychotherapy, New York, 1963, Harper & Row, Publishers.
7. Peplau, H.: Interpersonal techniques: the crux of psychiatric nursing, Am. J. Nurs. **62:** 50-54, 1962.
8. Ruesch, J.: Disturbed communication, New York, 1957, W. W. Norton & Co., p. 45.
9. Scheidlinger, S.: The relationship of group therapy to other group influence attempts. In Rosenbaum, M., and Berger, M. M., editors: Group psychotherapy and group function, New York, 1963, Basic Books, Inc., Publishers.
10. Schurman, M. J.: Five functions of the group therapist, Am. J. Nurs. **64:**108-110, 1964.
11. Yalom, I.: The theory and practice of group psychotherapy, New York, 1971, Basic Books, Inc., Publishers.
12. Yalom, I., and Terrazas, F.: Group therapy with chronic psychiatric patients, Modesto Hospital, Modesto, Calif., 1968. Unpublished manuscript.

SUGGESTED READINGS

Armstrong, J., and Rouslin, S.: Group psychotherapy in nursing practice, New York, 1963, The Macmillan Co.
Johnson, D. W., and Johnson, F. P.: Joining together—group therapy and group skills, Englewood Cliffs, N.J., 1975, Prentice-Hall, chap. 2.
Ullman, L., and Krasner, L.: Case studies in behavior modification, New York, 1965, Holt, Rinehart & Winston.
Wolpe, J., and Lazarus, A.: Behavior therapy techniques, New York, 1966, Pergamon Press.

CHAPTER 9

Establishing, maintaining, and terminating a group

Introduction

Establishing and maintaining a group experience for clients requires of the nurse certain knowledge and principles related to psychosocial adaptation and change in a small group setting. The nurse, with her unique focus on wellness, on explicit behavior change, and intelligent utilization of group interaction, as well as her supportive, facilitating style, can successfully conduct a group that supplements the efforts of her multidisciplinary team or provides the client with his primary source of restorative and preventive therapy.

The purpose of this chapter is to outline the specific tasks and principles necessary in the establishment, maintenance, and termination of the group experience.

The principles and considerations developed here are applicable to different kinds of groups (especially group psychotherapy and therapeutic groups with other than psychiatrically designated members). The reader will find these guide lines most useful in working with groups whose aim is promoting problem-solving behavior, facilitating more effective communication, and promoting insight.

Experiences with inpatient and outpatient groups and transition and supportive maintenance groups, as well as with couples and family group therapy, have been a major influence on me in specifying interventions and a theoretical perspective for this chapter.

The chapter is approached from an eclectic orientation, combining principles from analytic, interpersonal, communication, group process, and existential frameworks.

Appreciation is given to the idea that members symbolically reenact past relationships in the group, and these events effect the passage through phases, for example, termination. The interpersonal premise that anxiety arises from interpersonal interaction and is abated by establishing a safe place in the group is discussed as a task in the orientation phase of the group. The concept that members' communication patterns are indicative of interpersonal difficulties and are the target of change through a discussion of "here-and-now" communication in the group combines communication and Gestalt points of view. Lastly the group process premise that groups move through phases, and this fact suggests different interventions on the part of the group leader, is illustrated in the organization of the chapter as a whole.

In summary, this chapter joins some basic theoretical underpinnings with specific group stage-bound interventions that group leaders need to consider in establishing, maintaining, and terminating their group.

Group formation

The most important aspect of establishing a group is not locating where it will meet, deciding how many clients will be served, or deciding whether it should meet once or twice a week. Vital to the formative stage is the identification of the purpose and objectives of the group experience.

It is the purpose and objectives that determine all the beginning decisions about how many clients should be included and which clients should be asked to join. The purpose and objectives for a group are influenced by—

1. The theoretical background, philosophy, capabilities, and interests of the nurse
2. The characteristics of the client population accessible to the nurse
3. The requirements and goals of the agency employing the nurse
4. Any legal or professional standards that apply both to the private nurse practitioner and the nurse who is salaried by a public or private agency

The objectives of a group reflect both general and specific aims. They indicate the nurses' expectations of what benefit the group will serve its members and how, behaviorally, members' progress may be evaluated. For example, a general aim put forth in a couples therapy group I conducted was to increase the couples' awareness of their interpersonal communication patterns. But more specifically, I indicated my expectation that *each couple would recognize and describe for the group what communication pattern(s) they adopted when they disagreed about who was responsible for a decision.*

The following general aims of any group experience may be identified:

1. To enable members to gain greater knowledge of their behavior and relationships with others through feedback from members and leader(s) in a group setting
2. To provide reassurance and support through interpersonal contact in a group setting
3. To decrease members' sense of loneliness and feelings of isolation with their specific problem and thereby modify their feelings of powerlessness and hopelessness
4. To facilitate the opportunity for members to try out new, more successful communication patterns with others
5. To provide a safe environment where members can openly share their concerns and learn from the experiences of others in a group

Although there can be other aims the reader may identify, these goals are basic to any group experience and affect the leader's determination of specific objectives for members' participation. They also affect the nature of the nurse leadership role and what interventions will be indicated. To operationalize each of these aims the nurse must establish what outcomes in the group would provide certainty that the group was meeting its designed purposes. These overall aims of the group are then translated into more specific outcomes that enable the nurse to determine members' progress toward group goals.

In considering the first general aim of the group, we can identify several specific behaviors that serve as an index of this aim:

1. Members listen to one another when evaluative statements are made about their behavior in a given situation.
2. Members ask for clarification of the feedback they receive.
3. Members are able to describe what their intentions and expectations were behind their behavior.
4. Members are able to reflect on and describe the differences between their intentions and how their behavior was perceived by others.

Progress of the group toward fulfilling the second aim can be measured by the following behaviors:

1. Members are able to receive and value supportive gestures from other members and leader(s).
2. Members are able to express support and reassurance, when it is appropriate, to one another in the group.

The third general aim identified here was the ability to decrease members' feelings of loneliness and isolation. The following examples of members' behavior would indicate progress toward fulfilling this global expectation:

1. Members know the problems of one another (either superficially or in depth).
2. Members are able to identify how their problems, living situations, and stresses are like those of others in the group.
3. Members identify what aspects of a common problem were handled successfully by members in the group.

In order for the group to successfully facilitate members' trying out new communication patterns in the group, the following needs to occur:

1. Members become aware of what patterns they are currently using that are undesirable or unsuccessful.
2. Members identify alternative ways of communication as individuals communicate their needs in a manner that reflects their true thoughts and feelings.
3. Members use these alternatives in conversations with another person in the context of the group or outside the group setting.

Lastly, to provide a safe environment where open sharing can occur, members must—

1. Feel trust in the group and the leader(s) that what they say or do will be respected and not unduly held against them
2. Talk about and test out any fears they have about self-exposure
3. Develop increased ability to share all aspects of their concerns, including feelings and attitudes about events that worry or upset them

Once the nurse has clearly defined the overall goals of the group experience and has specified objectives or behavioral changes expected of members, and these logically relate to the goals, the selection of clients for the group can occur.

Screening and selecting members

Having become specific about the expectations for group members, the leader can judge more appropriately (1) who could benefit and (2) who is ready for this experience. Likewise, candidates who are informed of the objectives of the experience can take part in the decision as to whether they desire such a group experience.

It is true that the aims of a group imply who will fit and who will not, but the ability of the nurse to select certain clients who fit the objectives is sometimes limited. The nurse may find that the objectives for members may have to be modified to meet the needs of the people who are truly accessible. In this case the process of setting objectives is a fluid one in which the objectives determine who will belong and in which the characteristics of accessible clients influence what the objectives will be. The diagram below illustrates the interaction of objectives and accessible client characteristics.

This does not mean, however, that the leader gives up the aims of the group because members are unwilling to work toward some predetermined therapeutic purpose. If the leader does not take under consideration the level of psychological functioning of the clients and establish appropriate, attainable objectives (given what is possible for the group to achieve during the duration of the planned group experience), frustration will result, and the group will gain, under these circumstances, little therapeutic value from sessions. It is probable that members will view membership negatively, finding the attractiveness of the group dependent on pleasing the unrealistic expectations of the leader. Since cohesion may be lacking, premature termination is almost inevitable.

Important client characteristics. In deciding what client characteristics should be considered as important in the selection process, the nurse should have a working knowledge of the potential members as individuals. If the candidates for the group experience are hospitalized or are being seen by other health personnel in the agency, the nurse may have a great deal of indirect data from which to assess individuals. Care plans, nursing and medical records, the notes of other health professionals, and

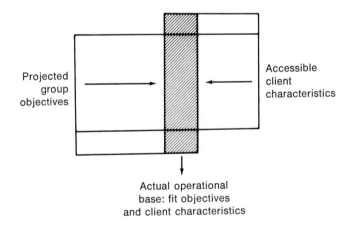

Projected group objectives

Accessible client characteristics

Actual operational base: fit objectives and client characteristics especially the histories taken by the health worker will be invaluable in gathering an impression of each candidate's strengths and indications for a group experience. This indirect information may not be enough, however, and one may choose to interview the client if he has been heretofore unfamiliar to the nurse, especially if a mental health assessment is not available.

A mental health assessment of each member should be completed. Whereas mental health status examinations to identify functional and emotional disorders in patients differ from institution to institution, there are some key categories common to all assessments that are essential to look at in interviewing individuals for possible group membership. The nurse should assess members'—

1. Affective or mood characteristics: What is the predominant mood of the member? Does it fluctuate? What extremes has the individual demonstrated? How will others' feelings influence the volatility of his mood fluctuation?
2. Thinking patterns: Does the member harbor illusions? Delusions? Does he hallucinate? Does he have ideas of reference? If so, what are his patterns and how is he likely to handle these in a group setting? Are his thoughts organized and coherent or are they disjointed and illogical? How would other members understand his communications in the group?
3. Interpersonal relationships: What are his chief ways of relating to other people around him, his family, friends, staff? What personal rewards might he get from his associations? In what areas would he avoid intimacy? For example, if he is hostile and aloof to staff and family, he may be resistant to giving and exchanging constructive feedback in the group. He may also block others' attempts to get to know him and understand his feelings.
4. Self-esteem and self-concept: How does he view himself? What does he see as his strengths and liabilities? How does he perceive himself in his roles, for example, of patient, employee, father, son, husband? How does he evaluate himself according to his perceptions of how he should be? How does he perceive how others see him? A patient's low self-esteem may cause him to assess all feedback, regardless of whether it is intended to be supportive or not, as critical and harsh.
5. Ego strength: What is his capacity to evaluate here-and-now experiences without distortion from past experiences? Can he check out his perception with other people or does he rely heavily on internal validation of his experience? For example, if the patient is autistic and validates stimuli chiefly through his own internal judgments, he will not be able to benefit as well from the aim of the group to increase insight through interpersonal feedback, and in this case a group with such a focus may be premature for him.
6. Communication patterns: What are his chief styles of communication? What does he communicate and what doesn't he? Does he communicate too much, too little, too late, too early, or in the wrong place, thereby making it difficult for others to understand him? How severe is his reliance on these patterns? If he has not achieved some ability to describe and state a reaction, thought, or experience, a process that develops in later childhood growth and develop-

ment, the group's expectations must include other means of facilitating expression of self that respect members' potentials and current liabilities.

When processing all the data about the potential member, the nurse needs to consider several general questions that will further help her decide the fit of the member for the group experience:

1. What are the client's strengths in sharing his experiences with others and appreciating others' problems?
2. What is the capacity of the client to tolerate feedback about his behavior?
3. How is the client currently handling interpersonal contact in the health care setting?
4. Are his problems sufficiently like those of other potential members so that he can benefit from mutual sharing and not feel "different" from others or deviant in the group?
5. If he has had therapeutic or therapy group experience before, were there certain positive outcomes realized by the client?

Authorities such as Yalom[5, p.156] and others agree that a client must be free of disruptive behavior in order to belong to a group and to get some worth of the experience and at the same time enable the group to proceed intact. Furthermore, Yalom[5, pp.157-158] explains that the brain-damaged, paranoid, suicidal, narcissistic, hypochondriacal, addicted, acutely psychotic, or sociopathic personalities are poor group risks. Yalom is describing those patients who are eligible for intensive outpatient group therapy. The nurse is not always in a position to rule out these patient categories but must be aware of how the group is shaping up in terms of numbers of patients categorized as disruptive. Therapeutic community groups and special problem groups, for example, are designed to meet the needs of some of these categories of clients, so it is unfair to charge that all these clients are poor group risks. In large part it depends on the group structure, the skills of the leader(s), and the group aims as to whether these clients are inappropriate group candidates. A more general and perhaps more useful criterion to the nurse who may function with a range of group modalities would be those assessment questions posed earlier.

If candidates are unable to participate in the activities and they become isolated and different in the group, then it is unlikely that they will get assistance and constructively support group aims. For example, if it occurs that group members are of widely divergent levels of psychological functioning, the group member who is functioning inadequately becomes an isolate. Such a group member may not be able to use what occurs in the group as a guide for increased functioning, and the formation of cohesiveness in the group may be prohibited.

The task of the group leader, then, is to strive for some degree of homogeneity in the group so that objectives will suit patient capacities and needs and members' personalities and problems will sufficiently match, so they can learn from one another without feeling isolated and estranged.

This is not to infer that heterogeneity is to be avoided. Differences in patients' coping styles and life experiences can facilitate learning from one another. However, if members cannot locate a basis of similarity in why they are in the group and what they have in common, they may deem their associations with each other as irrelevant and unnecessary. Locating commonalities between members promotes the feeling of homonymy that fosters beginning levels of group cohesiveness.

The criterion of "fit" in the group has been identified as a crucial factor in selection, but also in members' decisions to remain in the group or terminate early. Although the nurse may determine who will fit in the group, a client's feeling of belonging is individual and subjective. Clients may feel that they are different, that they do not belong, even though it is clear that they share similar problems with other members. Therefore an important step the leader should take is that of exploring with the candidate his expectations for the group and his perceptions of his needs. Usually candidates' perceptions are not articulated in the same manner as the objectives are defined. For example, patients may state that they want to know how other people solve their problems, want a place to go where people understand what it is like for them, or want to overcome a fear of talking in a group.

According to various studies of lay persons' perceptions of emotional disturbance and mental health, worrying, sadness, or inability to function as desired in a role may prompt people to seek help. These same motivations may be behind a client's choice of a group experience. The leader may recognize that it is possible to take these individual expectations and perceptions and translate them for the client so there is a better fit between the goals of the group as they have been specified and members' expectations of the benefits they will gain from their group experience.

Establishing a fit between group aims and members' perceptions and expectations is something the nurse can do in a pregroup interview with individuals when gathering selection data from the patient. It is possible while carrying out this task that the nurse will learn the degree of dissonance between members' perceptions and group aims.

If there is a great deal of variance after this discussion and the nurse decides, despite this fact, to include the individual in the group, then the success of the experience for the member may be severely limited. The client may resist verbal participation, avoid meetings, or focus the group discussion on the fact that he does not belong. This outcome is costly to the group and results in little growth in the client himself. What is more, the energy the nurse expends in trying to include him and handling his resistance will siphon off her effectiveness and capacity to deal with other group issues and other group interactions.

Some attention here must be given to the fact that the nurse will often be faced with the client who, in keeping with his psychological defense system, will deny the need for a group experience or will behave in the group inappropriately. For example, he may see that he has absolutely no problems or his ability to perform appropriate social behavior will be limited from time to time due to his high anxiety and autistic behavior. The nurse must weigh the advantages of including this member in the group, carefully assessing the effect this member will have and the predominance of the defense system.

It is highly recommended that the nurse not coerce any candidate to participate if he persists in not seeing the group experience as relevant or capable of meeting his needs at the time. Research[2] has indicated that the ability of the group to assist and influence an individual is contingent on whether he perceives the group as desirable. The ethical issue aside, nurses are wasting the client's, the group's, and their own time if they persist in including a member who does not fit the criteria nor accept the relevancy of the experience.

Yalom[5,pp.173–177] summarizes his opinion that clients are more likely to continue in group and therefore effectively benefit from their experience if they perceive the relevancy of the group experience in meeting their needs, can derive satisfaction from relationships with others and from participating in the tasks of the group, and take pride in belonging to the group.

Contracting for group membership

With group work, unlike working with individuals, there are three kinds of contracts the nurse must be aware of. One contract is that between leader and individual. Contracting means that the leader formulates a pact or agreement with a member for the achievement of objectives in the group meetings and for participation in the group. These objectives may be preformulated by the leader as mentioned earlier.

It is true that no member can commit himself to a group experience, or for that matter any other therapeutic experience, without understanding the purpose of the group, how the purpose is to be achieved, and what to expect from the therapeutic person. Vital to this understanding is a clear picture of what will be expected of him in order to meet the requirements of the group for participation and what requirements are imposed by personal goals in the group setting. Clients must be made aware of any risks to their participation and be assured by the leader that concrete steps are taken to modify any risks, real or imaginary. This particular aspect of the contract is sometimes dealt with on the implied level with clients' questioning the experience of the leader, why the leader is motivated to lead the group, and if the leader has received approval for the experience from agency authorities.

An agreement to participate requires members to have a basic sense of trust as well as readiness to get assistance for a problem. Yalom claims that the member must have faith in the omniscience of the leader. Above and beyond a patient's readiness is the importance of the sense of trust that leader extends to the client. The member is more likely to agree to a contract (1) if he perceives the leader as capable of producing desired results and (2) if he perceives the leader as biased in his behalf, that is, that the leader has the emotional and professional values to be client centered and can modify risks to him as an individual.

To summarize, then, before a client can commit himself to participate in the group, he must understand the purpose of the group, how the purpose is to be achieved, what is expected of him, and what he can expect from the leader. He must have the opportunity to reconstruct the group objectives in view of how he sees his needs. If these conditions are met and both leader and member are satisfied, then the contract is established sufficiently to proceed.

While the contract between leader and member is usually initiated at the first contact with the client, it may take more than one group session to fortify members' personal commitment. Inside the group the leader may reiterate the objectives and encourage members to share with one another their doubts, concerns, perceived needs, and preferences for the group. When the leader takes the business of the contract to the group, the nature of the contract extends to specify an agreement between the leader and group as a whole and members with one another. The leader is addressing the group in totality when speaking of objectives and conditions of participation. Members are also negotiating among themselves regarding which goals should take priority and what will be expected of one another to fulfill group aims.

The leader who does not recognize the importance of this aspect of the contract will misunderstand the impact of a group on individuals and the process of group problem solving. This beginning discussion between leader and group and between members regarding the contract will lay the foundation for the formulation of group norms. These beginning group norms may or may not support the identified aims of the group. It is vital that the leader act as goalkeeper and harmonizer in this beginning stage of negotiation. The leader must be aware that while the group is talking about the purposes of the group, they are in fact acting in a manner to support or deny these aims and may be testing the leader's ability to effectively keep the group together and direct the group discussion successfully. That is, they may be testing whether they can trust the leader, an essential ingredient if they are to agree to join the group and begin to take responsibility for their own participation.

In this beginning stage of contract formation the leader will understand that in the first several sessions of the group there is an implicit agreement made by members "to try it." In some cases the leader may verbalize explicitly that the group's attendance at these first sessions indicates that they have given tentative agreement to meeting together, although all aspects of the experience are not clear to them yet and the group has not had a chance to discuss all the objectives of the experience. The group's continuance is proof that the group perceives a basis for common problems and goals and trusts the leader to some extent. It is important that the leader acknowledge with the group, when they have had sufficient time to discuss the objectives for the group, that continued attendance and participation is interpreted by her to mean that there is a consensus in the group to work toward the ends discussed. Whereas some groups may take an explicit vote to accept an agenda, this procedure may not occur. However, it is important that the leader verbalize the implied nature of consensus, earmarking an important landmark in the group's developmental process.

Structuring the group experience

With every group experience there should be a discrete organizational structure that facilitates group goals. Considerations such as how many members should be included, where the group should meet, whether it should be an open or closed group, and what should be the duration of sessions and duration of the entire group experience must be reviewed in light of group aims and basic considerations about group development.

Size. It is understood that the usual size of a small group for therapeutic purposes should be six to ten individuals plus the leader. Although the leader may include one or two extras in the group in case someone drops out, and the aim is to have a closed group for a certain time period, it is felt that any more (or less) in the group will inhibit the kind of feedback exchange desired to promote client self-awareness.

It is noted by many leaders that a group of four or fewer persons does not operate as a group unless it is a residential or family group. The leader may not feel it worthwhile to offer a group experience due to the fact that it is like conducting a one-to-one relationship with three or four people at the same time. There are fewer opportunities for members to stimulate each other's reactions and a tendency toward conversation with the leader versus exchange among members. Yalom indicates that as a group's size diminishes, the advantages of the group experience, for example, the opportunity to interact with a variety of individuals and get a variation in feedback, is limited.

The upper limit of a group's size is also contingent on the objectives of the group experience. Although Yalom and others indicate that size prohibits working through of individual problems, it must be noted that there are several innovative approaches to group work currently practiced that successfully counteract the barrier of size.

EST (Erhard Seminar Training), for example, conducts group experiences with 250 people at a time. EST takes several measures to enforce community pressure to change, to provide for consensual validation, and to ensure that members work on their own individual problems. The placement of chairs, verbal feedback to the group, and reinforcement for sharing and truth processes directed by the group leader successfully handle many of the heretofore barriers small group leaders saw in conducting large group sessions. The questions arise as to what are the skills of the client group in coping with the objectives and structure of the group and what are the particular leader's abilities that would dictate a maximum number of members of more than six to ten persons.

There are reasons why a group may be limited to traditional group size. If group members vary in ability to cope with anxiety, and some members need external encouragement to seek out and give feedback in a group, the leader would have a rationale to limit the size of the group to the traditional therapeutic model. Also, if the leader is a novice, or is uncomfortable with large numbers of clients whom he cannot readily see or assess their response, the smaller group format may address his need for control in the group.

There is definitely a need for the leader, as an expert in interpersonal relationships and with something important to contribute in the context of viewing group members' transactions, to intervene in the group and direct others in testing alternative ways of interacting with one another. The small group format is perhaps still most facilitative of here-and-now analysis of interpersonal communication processes.

In a study by Castore[1] regarding the impact of size on member-to-member exchange, a marked reduction in interactions between members was found when the group had nine members and a second clear reduction when the group's size was 17 or more members. This study implied that for inpatient therapy groups the ideal size would be five to eight persons if patients were to benefit from maximum client-to-client interchange.

It is important to note that this research was done with therapy groups only and probably had a traditional basis of operation to facilitate member exchange. Although it holds important implications for consideration for size, and most group leaders would support the dictum of five to eight persons, it does not apply to every group modality. There are ways to overcome the disadvantages of a large group, and the nurse is frequently in a position to work with other than the ideal size. In psychiatric community meetings, consciousness-raising groups, and therapeutic and patient education groups with other than psychiatric clients, the nurse may be expected to operate with large numbers of individuals. Instead of developing a "fixed idea" about the maximum number of clients desirable, it is better that the nurse judge size on the basis of specific group objectives and on client abilities to utilize group feedback and that she know how to work with the barriers that sometimes arise from larger group constellations.

When the nurse is leading a "captive" group, that is, designated numbers of individuals that are required to attend, the matter of size will only be one barrier to the group's effective interaction. The fact that some patients do not choose to be there, and thus individually resist group feedback, may be a more reliable predictor of their interaction with one another than the sheer number of individuals present.

Ideal setting. There are many principles the nurse should consider when selecting the ideal place and time for a group experience. The ideal place for a group setting is one that promotes members' feelings of safety and security in the group. Deciding on what environment will address this principle requires the nurse to know and anticipate the various fears and concerns of the clients. The time and place of the meeting are within the domain of group leadership decisions and should produce no particular barriers to members or leader. The time of the meeting should fit the members' schedules sufficiently to limit conflicts in commitments and allow them to arrive on time and leave at the scheduled time. The meeting place should be accessible to everyone and must be available for the specified time period throughout the duration of the group.

Confidentiality and privacy are basic concerns of most members. Therefore the nurse should choose a room that preserves the sense of group privacy and not an area of an agency that exposes the group to distracting interruptions from others who they fear will criticize or reject them if they heard what is being talked about. Although the setting must assure client and group privacy, it must not be so enclosed that it creates undue anxiety in patients who fear they cannot control their own impulses or that they may be harmed by other patients in the group. A clear route to the exit and sufficient spaces between chairs may be comforting to patients whose chief concern is intimacy in a group and who fear that they may act out unacceptable impulses.

The ideal place for a group should also promote a positive, open exchange between members. One nurse who had chosen what she thought was an ideal private room to hold a meeting was dismayed when she found the session resulted in very little discussion by patients and a "tense" atmosphere. Although this session was the first meeting, and tension is generally high in the beginning, it was noted that the interior of the room probably contributed to the resistance in the group. The room was small, there were no ashtrays, and patients had only hardback chairs. The walls were a drab gray blue, and except for a chart on the wall there were no particular wall fixtures or appealing design. The same nurse noted a difference in her own enthusiasm and the participation of others in a different group in another office space. This office was no larger but had brighter lighting, padded chairs, and wall decorations. Although the patients were similarly regressed and withdrawn in behavior, there seemed to be an affectively different experience for patients and leader in the second group—one of more openness and willingness to be together. The difference in attractiveness of the two rooms may have had an effect on patient and leader attitudes.

Duration. The duration of each session and of the entire group experience is a problem with which nurses have not traditionally had to deal. Like the selection of clients and the composition of the group, this decision has in the past been made as a consequence of treatment regimen and physician preference. An agency may have established a standard for the length of experience, or the psychiatrist may have decided the length and intensity of a group experience for his client. If the nurse is a junior coleader in the group, she may or may not have been brought into decisions about the duration of the group experience. More and more, however, nurses are being asked to decide the intensity and duration of therapeutic experience for the patient. Therefore it is important for the nurse to be aware of some overall principles in deciding how long the meetings should last and what is a desirable length for the life of the group.

The hours of a group are a constant in the experience and are part of the group contract. If a group is designed to meet from 10:00 to 11:30 AM every Monday and Wednesday and the leader and members do not adhere to this time prescription either by showing up late or going overtime, a violation of the contract has occurred. Likewise, if the group disbands in 2 months when the agreement was that it would meet for a minimum of 6 months, or extends past the 6-month period, the group aims have been forfeited or modified, and it is important that both the members and leaders realize the basis for this infringement on the contract.

It is often the case with beginning leaders that they do not understand the importance of meeting as prescribed, and in an attempt to cope with this conflict, for example, pleasing members, they may not hold the group to the agreed on schedule. Since the time schedule of the group is a matter of the contract, and group adherence demonstrates group success, the leader must not regard time considerations casually. Members rely on the leader to set an example and look to the structure of the group as something they can trust. If the leader is disrespectful of this aspect of the group, she is setting herself up to be seen as insincere and unreliable. Any advantage the leader may have hoped to achieve by way of appearing "flexible" and "loose" has been lost to patient frustration and doubt.

Of late there are many variations in the length of group sessions. The intensity of human experience desired and the leader's perceptions of the skills and limitations of members, as well as the goals of the group, will guide decisions of this kind. Although the most common approach is for a group to be held once or twice a week for 1 to 1½ hours each time, this format may vary drastically. If an exchange of human feelings among neurotic individuals with the result of increased awareness of fears of intimacy is the case, the nurse may choose a marathon experience for the group. Marathons or time-extended groups are ongoing, uninterrupted group experiences, lasting anywhere from 6 hours (the minimarathon) to a whole weekend (up to 24 or more hours) in residence. Marathons may be used to assist relatively well individuals to gain increased awareness of self and others and of group dynamics. The advantages of the marathon approach are many. It speeds up group development and intensifies members' emotional experience as well as facilitates more authentic feedback between members about their "real" fears, thoughts, and feelings.

Despite the positive attributes associated with the marathon group, the time intensity experience has been looked at with suspicion and has not been accepted as a format for acutely psychotic or chronically disturbed individuals. As pointed out in Part One of this text, time intensity experiences tend to strip members of defense mechanisms in an attempt to produce more authentic interrelating. Maintenance of defenses, such as blocking recollection of unpleasant experiences and avoidance of feelings that are highly emotionally charged due to former life experiences, is often encouraged in the psychotic person who cannot differentiate whether he has or will act on unacceptable desires. Likewise a time-intense experience has not been widely utilized by special problem groups. In problem-focused groups, continuity of support is felt to be essential; the emphasis is on behavior change achieved through reinforcement of desirable traits and goals. Single, isolated episodes of relinquishing undesirable behavior in a highly intense interaction is not sustaining enough for members interested in long-term coping and irreversible behavior change.

To determine the exact duration of the total group experience, the nurse is best guided by the objectives of the experience and, at best, an experienced and educated guess about how long the group will need to take care of its tasks. The nurse may arbitrarily set a duration at the outset, for example, for 3 months twice a week for 1½ hours. It is generally thought that it takes at least 5 therapeutic contact hours for the group to reach a working phase and that in some cases it may be as much as 12 hours. This means that the group needs not less than four sessions to arrive at a working phase. The working phase may extend as long as it takes to meet the objectives, and termination requires at least two to three sessions if the issue of separation is to be handled with satisfaction. In most instances, with exceptions such as crisis-oriented, short-term group psychotherapy, the group experience should extend beyond eight sessions, each session lasting 1½ hours.

It is my observation that with this format the group can achieve general aims within a 3-month period and work more specifically on changing individual behavior if the group has a 6-month life. It is the reaction of many of my students who are confined to their semester course schedule that at the time they are ending their group they are "just getting started," that members are just beginning to test out new behaviors, and that the group is just beginning to learn from the interaction and feedback they receive in the group.

Phases of group experience

It is a generally well-accepted premise that the life of a group can be viewed in three distinct phases or stages. In psychotherapeutic terminology these phases are the introductory or beginning phase, the working-through or middle phase, and the termination phase. While theorists differ in their conceptions of the subphases of groups, usually depending on their theoretical framework, the majority concede that these phases exist and call for different functioning and considerations on the part of the group leaders.

Phase I. The introductory phase: securing a psychosocial environment conducive to self-expression

Once objectives are established, members are screened, and an adequate environment for assemblage of the group is arranged, it is the task of the group leader to create an atmosphere of interpersonal safety that will promote self-expression and build cohesiveness.

It is one thing to attend to the physical features of the group setting and the organizational parameters of the group experience, but quite another to create an interpersonal exchange that facilitates self-disclosure. A clear design for the group and pleasant surroundings will promote members' sharing of thoughts and feelings, but the skill of the leader in creating interpersonal safety and mobilizing constructive group norms is vital.

Self-disclosure occurs when one person voluntarily tells another things about himself that the other is unlikely to know or discover from other sources.

Jourard[3] and others have stressed the fact that self-disclosure leads to knowledge of self and is an important goal of the therapeutic process in a group or other client contact situations. To promote member self-disclosure the nurse must be able to instill trust. By trust is meant the belief that the nurse is capable of handling members' behavior and capable of assisting members to achieve the aims of the group. At least for the first sessions of the group the nurse is the goalkeeper. It is the nurse's responsibility to assist the group in clarifying objectives and incorporating individual idiosyncratic needs into the total group framework. By serving as goalkeeper the nurse fortifies members' confidence in the leader and the group as a viable therapeutic modality. By acknowledging members' respective needs the nurse demonstrates a bias toward each member and an ability to accept the members as they are.

These steps in the process of establishing a psychosocial environment conducive to self-disclosure are further enhanced by the attitude and nonverbal communication of the nurse. Conveying acceptance, understanding, and a positive attitude toward members' contributions—no matter how inappropriate some contributions may appear—will encourage members to regard the group as a safe place.

These interventions must also be delivered in a framework of appropriate norm setting. Norms that foster group safety and support group goals are negotiated at the beginning of each group. Sometimes the nurse will express these norms overtly to the group, for example, "It is essential that everyone participate by sharing their experiences;" or "Members should allow each person to finish speaking before he interjects his opinions." These norms become ground rules for members' participation in the group. Standards, for example, to work on problems and avoid extraneous conversation or to avoid retaliating when someone criticizes you in the group, are norms as well but may be covert rules in the group that are not established and voiced by the nurse at the outset.

The nurse leader must be alert to the impact of the ground rules she imposes on the group and those that the group establishes by way of members' subsequent interaction with one another. If the ground rules she imposes threaten members or if the norms formed in the course of the group prevent members from reaching group objectives, she must stop the process and reexamine the covert standards established for group interaction.

Beginning covert conflicts in the group may emerge around specific fears about sharing problems, being singled out by the leader, getting close to others, and mixing with other emotionally traumatized members. While members may fear these situations, they may have equally compelling needs to get help from the leader and feel included in the group. The nurse must be aware of these conflicts and how they affect achievement of group goals. She must provide support for the expression of these fears and reinforce solutions that promote safe self-disclosure in the group. The nurse should understand that the movement and progress of the group is a result of how the group resolves these and subsequent conflicts about intimacy, authority, and change.

Clients' trust in the leader will diffuse to the group in general, provided members learn successfully how to handle group issues and are secure in the confidentiality of group business. Confidentiality is established by the group when members agree to handle self-disclosure with discretion. This means that members should agree not to reveal what has been said outside the group and that what is said will not be unduly held against a member inside the group. Without this basic reassurance, members cannot feel free to divulge thoughts and feelings that they themselves judge as crazy, abnormal, or otherwise painful. For the most part, confidentiality of group business can be achieved by a statement of the leader or by an open discussion of the group.

Usually the leader has already conveyed this expectation during the assessment interview; this discussion by the group is additional support to a critical group feature.

The real test of the group's ability to handle group issues will come with member interaction. How members trust one another, their ability to meet group goals, and leader expectations will be evaluated on the basis of "trial balloons." Such a trial balloon may be determining what the group should talk about or how the group will give feedback to a member. The outcome of these group tasks will contribute to or deter from the confidence and trust members instill in the group and in themselves to get better through the group experience.

Phase II. The working phase: locating responsibility in members for change

If the members have established a mutual sense of trust and confidence in the group as well as in the leader, real working on problems can occur. This stage of the group will also be evident in that members will have a clearer picture of other members as unique persons, will understand more precisely what is appropriate and necessary to work on in the group, and can accept, at least at a beginning level, feedback from others.

This phase marks the genuine beginning of members' ability to focus on specific problems and locate responsibility for these problems in themselves. They will accept the idea that they may not be able to communicate effectively or that they are afraid of criticism, for example, and will begin to experiment with different ways of behaving in the group and outside the group setting.

Generally members can tolerate feedback without resisting all possibility that they are at fault or that the feedback may have credibility. They can tolerate this responsibility because they have a basis of trust and confidence in the group. It is in this phase of the group that the leader will experience some relaxation of the need to actively direct the group discussion, call for feedback from members, and ask members to share. I have described aspects of this phase of the group as aspects of putting the group on "automatic pilot." That is, the group members will initiate verbal exchange directed toward shared experiences and assume various leadership activities that give the nurse the impression that very little else has to be done to move the group to important insights or expected outcomes. The open exploration of feelings, attitudes, and behaviors enables members to compare and contrast their experiences in and outside of the group situation.

At this time they are open to new generalizations about relationships and can explore new ways of gaining support and solving dilemmas. This point is illustrated by one therapeutic group with stroke patients that moved from a hesitant attitude of looking at problems to an open, realistic confrontation of their problems.

In the first stage they talked unrealistically about discharge plans, denying the realities of their limitations. With supportive leadership they were able to come to terms with aspects of their altered role in their family and community. By providing members space to vent feelings of frustration and anger in the first stage the leaders promoted self-disclosure and cohesion; this in turn supported the movement of members to identify new ways of coping with restrictions due to their stroke experiences. This movement was voluntary and clearly a chosen direction of the group.

The apparent ease of the group in handling problems and group discussion is intermixed, however, with periodic individual resistances and group blocking. This is a result of members' feeling powerless over their problems where responsibility for their thoughts, feelings, and behavior is too burdensome or painful. As the group learns of one another's problems, members may be eager to confront and solve what seems to be obvious barriers in individuals' lives. What it has not counted on is that members have a stake in feelings and behavior they have harbored, no matter how destructive these feelings or behavior is to their general well-being.

Confrontation with one another may result in members' employing various defense mechanisms to avoid change. These mechanisms may include missing group meetings, attacking the group when one is being confronted, or a sudden lapse in memory. For example, one member in a psychotherapy group could not remember what the group had told her about her offensive sarcasm during the previous meeting. She went so far as to claim that she did not say what the group thought she had said. This denial and forgetting process enabled her to temporarily block out the realization that she may be a very hostile person, something that was totally opposite to her desired self-image. Instead of working on changing her sarcastic behavior through the realization of her hostility, the patient denied her anger and resumed her sarcasm in a one-upmanship position in the group: "You are reading things into what I said; no one ever knows how I feel."

The resistance in the working phase of the group is almost always due to the fact that members are running headlong into the self they feared they were and of which they were not aware or of which they were keeping to themselves. We can utilize Johari's[4] diagram to illustrate this point. There are at least four aspects of the self the client experiences. These are (1) that part of the self with which he and others are aware, (2) the self with which he is not aware of and others are aware, (3) the self with which he is aware but others are not, and (4) the self with which neither the client nor others are aware.

Client aware; others not	Client aware; others are
Others aware; client is not	Others not aware; client not aware

In the first phase of the group the group is dealing with material that is non-threatening—that which the clients can acknowledge about themselves in front of themselves and others. During the middle phase of the group there is a greater probability that members will experience that part of themselves with which they were formerly aware and which others were not aware of but have grown to know, or they may be confronted with what they were not aware of but is discernible by the group. Also, because of the increased level of intimacy in the group, members are more likely to develop transference of feelings, thoughts, and behavior to the group and leader from former life experiences. This transference process allows members to gain greater awareness of how they distort present situations in terms of past events and what areas of human interaction trigger their emotional difficulties. This new data, personal in nature, can contribute to the anxiety and discomfort of individuals and block their movement toward change and the group's ability to assist them. But at the same time it can open up opportunities for interpersonal learning to occur.

The following example illustrates how one member achieved greater insight into her personal interactions with the leader. This member, after two sequential absences of the leader, charged, "You don't care about us—you are too busy with other things."

Instead of becoming defensive and justifying her absences, the leader asked if this "not caring" was something other members picked up. Some replied "no" but supported the verbal charge by explaining, "I can understand why Judy feels the way she does." The leader claimed that maybe Judy's concern was not fully explored yet.

Through the process of having Judy restate her feelings and describe specifically what bothered her, she was able to identify that she felt this way before—that she felt left alone a great deal by her parents and was expecting that her husband would soon separate from her and her children, leaving her "helpless." She saw that the leader's cancellation of sessions made her afraid that there would be absolutely no support for her when she really needed it. Her anger at the leader was generated out of fear and frustration that she could not help herself and get the support from others that she needed.

The attitude of the leader and the group's permission to work through former problems through present group relationships will be crucial to members' ability to work on these personality features. Usually the understanding and acceptance of the group will ease the tension experienced and assist members in working on and reexamining those parts of themselves deemed desirable and undesirable. It is likely that the group will be more lenient in its judgment than the member himself and enable the member to accept a new level of responsibility for his behavior and feelings. In some cases members will share that they have had the same uncomfortable insights, and this will serve as further group support to individuals who are facing these problems for the first time or reexperiencing former fears.

Therapeutic problem solving can best be achieved in the working phase because of the tendency for relevant material to arise as group business and the ability of the group to offer support. Real and fantasized problems that concern the patient may be identified. Needs for change may be realized via feedback from others. Alternatives can be discussed because the problems are shared, and commitment to try out new behaviors is tolerated by the added awareness of the individual regarding the impact of his problem and the group's commitment to bettering the experience of its member.

For example, in one group a member grew to learn that her own dependency on her spouse was having detrimental effects on their relationship and her own sense of powerfulness. The group encouraged her to stand up for her preferences and let her spouse know when she needed something and wanted freedom to make her own decision. The member experimented with this change and reported to the group instances in which she did communicate her individuality to others. This feedback to the group reinforced the member's attempts to change and was useful to the group as a whole.

When a group member attempts a change, success is individually assigned but felt by the group. The group may feel as much pride as the individual who has achieved the change. Likewise the group's ability to help one member has individual meaning for each and every one of the members. Knowing that you are a part of the group that helped someone get better reinforces your own sense of self-worth and dignity.

The leader can serve an important function in group success by reinforcing the individual's attempts to change. Inviting him to try out a change inside the group, encouraging the group to report on the change they see, and showing interest in how the change has worked on the outside will reinforce members' sense of responsibility and power to make their life better through group involvement.

Phase III. Terminating the group: arriving at a perspective on self and others through change

The tasks of this final phase of the group are to summarize the experience, establish perspective, and bring closure to the group. The leader focuses on identifying the impact the group has had on each member and assists herself and others to confront the experience of loss generated by the termination of the group experience.

It is perhaps rare indeed that all groups end when they should, and even more so, that all members continue in the group until it is indicated that they have nothing more to gain. The drop-out rate of individuals in groups is still significantly high. The focus of this discussion, however, is on knowing when the clients and the group have benefited to the maximum.

If the leader has sufficiently identified the outcomes of the group experience and has operationalized these outcomes in a way that some determination may be made about success, then the decision about when to terminate the group is self-explanatory. Therefore the nurse will want to be as clear as possible at the outset as to the criteria for group success. The nurse may use a number of means to evaluate the progress of the group. Group members' verbal assessments of the group are one source of data that should not be ignored. Members' behavior in and outside the group in other social or living groups is another indicator of client movement. The assessments of other staff and agency informants are still another source of data.

In addition to the criteria established by the specific group's objectives and contract, which established a designated period for group life, the nurse may rely on some general landmarks that will give her further support for terminating the group. One criterion is whether the member feels that he has gotten as much out of the group as possible. He may indicate this through his quick insight, his ability to alter his problematic behavior, and his feelings of being able to manage his life. These are not transitory feelings but attitudes arrived at after seriously working on problems and coming to some resolution of conflicts experienced in the group. The group as a whole may show signs of boredom and turn more to a socializing group, symbolizing there is no more work to do.

Because groups do not always end as a result of a systematic assessment of group growth, it is important to consider other reasons why groups terminate. If the group is set up in an inpatient setting and is not an open-ended group, the group may terminate when the majority of the members are discharged due to physician-perceived progress on their present symptoms. Still another reason may be patients' lack of continual attendance to the point that the group is no longer viable. Whatever the reasons for termination, anticipated and planned or unpredictable and somewhat sudden, it is important that the leader provide adequate opportunity to bring closure on group issues.

Like termination of a significant one-to-one relationship, termination of group relationships can arouse feelings of anxiety and loss that lead to temporary episodes of regression in some members. The leader should provide sufficient opportunity for members to express their feelings and gain perspective about their separation from the group, the leader, and individual members. The leader is obliged to bring up the subject of group termination at least 2 to 3 weeks in advance of the last session, depending on the duration, how frequently the group meets, and how intense the experience has been. The nurse may stimulate self-disclosure of feelings about termination through various means, including communicating her own feelings about the group terminating and what the group has meant to her.

Depending on the intensity of members' feelings of loss and the degree to which loss is a former psychological trauma to members, the leader may be tempted to equate the experience of loss of the group with the loss of others in the past. Whereas this discussion may stimulate insight in patients about their current reactions, the nurse must be aware of the risk she is taking in deliberately raising issues from the past. If the nurse does not have the time to help patients work through what painful memories arise, or if she feels she does not have the skill to deal effectively with this material, then it is best that she focus exclusively on the here and now, what feelings members have about this group and this termination experience.

Termination is a time to take stock of group progress and to generally evaluate the experience. Where group work is one modality in a sequence of subsequent treatment programs, the nurse should help the members evaluate what progress they have made in the group and what problems they need to focus on in other aspects of the program or in the future in general. If the nurse conveys the philosophy that the achievement of mental health and growth is a continuous process, then members are less likely to concede that the group was a failure because it did not solve all their problems or that they will never need emotional counseling again. This point of view of progressing toward greater health and growth via stages is likely to make members more cooperative with other phases of their treatment program and curtail the formulation of grandiose ideas about their abilities to master their life and change the world after group termination.

It is well publicized that self-growth groups, for example, generate a "high" based on the group's achievement of greater self insights and more effective interpersonal communication. A member who graduates from this experience may decide that he can alter his work, family, or community relationships in a fashion parallel to the group's achievements. The reality of his powerlessness, which comes to him shortly after his feelings of mastery, can either cause him to discredit what he learned in the group or consider himself a failure in producing social change.

For this reason many self-awareness group formats provide for a gradual weaning process and one or two post-termination sessions to talk about the emotional letdown members may be experiencing. These sessions, usually one or two at the most, may be scheduled 1 or 2 weeks after the group terminates. The leader is careful about resuming group life for other than transition purposes.

The concept of gradual weaning from the group is a good one and can be executed in all groups. The leader may decrease the time of the session or the frequency of the meetings. She may also interject socializing activities near the termination date that allow members to pull away from the intensity of working on problems and help members bring symbolic closure to the group.

The leader must be aware that because separation and loss do generate many painful feelings in many members, the group and individuals within the group, as well as herself, may resist dealing with the issue. The group may cope by avoiding discussions about termination, denying that they have feelings, and denying the importance to them of the group and leader. The leader may feel anxious about discussing separation, feel pangs of guilt, for example, that the group did not handle everything it could or may disengage emotionally from the group. Outside support from the nurse's supervisor will help her in becoming more aware of her own reactions to group termination. Individual members may act out their resistance by regressing, terminating their attendance prematurely, changing the subject inside the group, or insisting that the group must continue. A group that has had a great number of positive affectual experiences may collaborate to continue group meetings past the designated termination date.

It is the nurse's responsibility to assess the reactions of herself and the group, to acknowledge these reactions, and to help the group examine why they are resorting to these behaviors. If the nurse examines the wish or fear behind these reactions, then both she and the group will be freed of holding to these behaviors and can more comfortably let go of the group.

When the fears of the group revolve around survival (for example, How will I live without the group?), the nurse must point out the realities of the situation; for example, that they have survived before the group and will survive without the group and that the group, while seemingly powerful in their lives at the moment, was not always viewed in this way. Ultimately they alone have the responsibility for their survival—something they have taken on in the past but which may seem overwhelming to them at the moment when they realize they will no longer be coming to the group.

REFERENCES

1. Castore, G. F.: Number of verbal interrelationships as a determinant of group size, J. Abnorm. Psychol. **64:**456-457, 1962.
2. Festinger, S., Schacter, S., and Boch, K.: The operation of group standards. In Cartwright, D., and Zander, A.: Group dynamics—research and theory, ed. 3, New York, 1968, Harper & Row, Publishers, pp. 241-259.
3. Jourard, S. M.: Healthy personality, New York, 1974, The Macmillan Co.
4. Luft, J., and Ingham, H.: The Johari window: a graphic model of interpersonal awareness, Proceedings of the Western Training Laboratory in Group Development, Los Angeles, 1955, University of California Extension Office.
5. Yalom, I. D.: The theory and practice of group psychotherapy, New York, 1970, Basic Books, Inc., Publishers.

SUGGESTED READINGS

Burgess, A. W., and Lazare, A.: Psychiatric nursing in the hospital and the community, Englewood Cliffs, N.J., 1976, Prentice-Hall, pp. 185-199.

Janosik, E. H.: A pragmatic approach to group therapy, J. Psychiatr. Nurs. **10:**7-11, 1972.

Johnson, D. L., and Gold, S. R.: An empirical approach to issues on selection and evaluation in group therapy, Int. J. Group Psychother. **21:**321-339, 1971.

Loomis, M. E., and Dodenhoff, J. T.: Working with informal patient groups, Am. J. Nurs. **70:**1939-1944, 1970.

McGrew, L., and Jensen, J. L.: A technique for facilitating therapeutic group interaction, J. Psychiatr. Nurs. **10:**18-21, 1972.

Pearce, W. B., and Sharp, S. M.: Self-disclosing communication, J. Commun. **23**(4):409-425, 1973.

Smith, A. J.: A manual for the training of psychiatric nursing personnel in group psychotherapy, Perspect. Psychiatr. Care **8:**107-126, 1970.

Sweeney, A., and Draze, E.: Group therapy—an analysis of the orientation phase, J. Psychiatr. Nurs. **6:**20-26, 1968.

Wenburg, J. R., and Wilmont, W. W.: The personal communication process, New York, 1973, John Wiley & Sons.

Yalom, I.: The theory and practice of group psychotherapy, New York, 1970, Basic Books, Inc., Publishers.

CHAPTER 10

Group practice and empirical observations—some case studies

Introduction

In this chapter we will describe several group situations in which the nurse might choose to operate as a group leader or group therapist. The case studies presented here illustrate various types of groups, from therapy groups to self-growth groups. We do not, by any means, attempt to give an illustration of every type of group in which the nurse may choose to operate. These case studies provide the reader with an insight into how nurses may operate in different groups, specific problems that may arise due to the types of clients in the group and the purposes of the group, and how nurses can employ various theoretical frameworks, for example, communication, analytic, interpersonal relationship, and group dynamics theories, to guide their perceptions of the group and their selection of interventions.

In each of the six case studies presented here I have chosen to focus specifically on certain problems and to employ interventions that fit a particular theoretical framework. My choice of problems to focus on in each group reflects a certain problem-solving process. Before I accepted the role of leader in these groups, I had a sound knowledge of my own capabilities as a group leader and of my attitudes toward people and their problems, as well as of the interpersonal handicaps I might have in relating to others. I was generally aware of the strengths and limitations of members and of what they might reasonably work on in the time allotted for their group experience. The first two sessions of a group I spent assessing to a greater extent the concerns of members and how the group might be beneficial. I also became aware of what problems would arise to affect the cohesiveness of the group and its ability to provide members with a sense of belongingness, companionship, and security. Although I could view the groups as having more than one possible effect on members, I chose to confine my focus to a certain area, which was paramount if members were to grow individually and essential if the group was to provide the general benefits of group membership. In one instance I chose to focus on dysfunctional communication syndromes; in another I chose to look at the group focal conflicts as they were manifested in the group. In these two cases I selected very different theoretical foundations by which to view the problems of the group and guide my interventions. My selection of a theoretical framework was greatly influenced by the problems individuals manifested in the group and also by the theories that seemed best in explaining phenomena in the group and that would promote the selection of appropriate interventions.

The following case studies illustrate the nurse group leader's selection of a specific focus and certain theoretical bases to guide her perceptions and interventions in the group. These studies illustrate how some of the theoretical frameworks discussed in Chapter 6 might be employed in actual practice situations and how the nurse might function in some of those groups outlined in Part One.

Case study 1. Dysfunctional communication syndromes in a married couples group*

Dysfunctional communication syndromes become integrated into systems of many unhealthy couples' interactions. These syndromes may or may not be necessary for continuation of the couples' relations but often serve the purpose of increasing one partner's self-esteem at the cost of the other's feelings of self-worth and at the cost of effective communication per se. Two syndromes seemed to prevail in a married couples group I led over a period of 6 months. These were the "blame" or "If only you . . . " syndrome and the "mind-reading" syndrome. We will describe these syndromes as they emerged in the group and examine the role of the nurse group therapist in (1) discouraging the use of these syndromes, (2) helping members to develop further insight as to their communication patterns, and (3) helping members to adopt more functional ways of communicating—the major objectives of this group experience.

The married couples group depicted here is a group of four to five couples seen by the nurse once a week for 1½ hours in a veteran's administration mental hygiene clinic. In each case the husband had been previously hospitalized for emotional illness; in three cases the wife, too, had either been hospitalized or had received private psychiatric help or clinic services for emotional problems.

The syndromes

Several dysfunctional communication syndromes[10] seemed to be operating in this group. Those syndromes that were most prevalent were the blame and the mind-reading syndromes. With the blame or "If only you . . . " syndrome, spouse 1 asks for change in the other, spouse 2, by complaining. Because this technique suggests that spouse 1 is "blameless," he is relieved of responsibility for change. He is portrayed favorably to the rest of the group at the cost of making his mate appear at fault. Spouse 2 may feel anxious, angry, or guilty; to save face she may disclaim spouse 1's accusations and counter likewise: "If you would just . . . then I could . . . " A tit-for-tat system results whereby both partners deny that change involves a joint effort, and much of the communication that follows is not heard, not qualified, misunderstood, or ignored.

The following is an example of how Joe and Nadine participated in the blame

---

*Modified from paper presented by Marram, G. D., at the Tenth Annual Conference of the Golden Gate Group Psychotherapy Society, San Francisco, June 13-14, 1969.

syndrome, indicating among other things how these syndromes serve to increase one partner's self-esteem at the cost of the other's feelings of self-worth and at the cost of effective communication.

NURSE: What do you see your problem to be, Joe and Nadine?

JOE: If she would just sit down and talk with me . . . we could get things worked out . . . (complaining tone of voice)

NADINE: (interrupts Joe) It won't work, Joe. I've never been able to sit down and talk with you because you . . . (accusing tone of voice)

JOE: (silent, hurt expression on his face)

NURSE: What are you thinking, Joe?

JOE: It's useless . . . I can't change her mind. (pause) Things would be okay if only she'd be willing to sit down and discuss our problems.

Joe in this case asks for change in Nadine by complaining. At the same time he suggests that Nadine and her unwillingness to talk constitute a problem for the two. Joe portrays himself as "blameless" and in doing so relieves himself of responsibility for change. He appears favorably to the rest of the group because, unlike Nadine, he apparently wants to work toward a solution to their problems. Nadine is made to seem at fault. In an attempt to save face she claims that Joe does not have the answer, that is, "It won't work . . . ," and counters likewise, suggesting that Joe's behavior is the reason they have not been able to sit down and talk. In turn she too has relieved herself of blame and responsibility for change. Both Joe and Nadine have trouble in acknowledging that change involves a joint effort. If the nurse had not interrupted to ask Joe about what he was thinking, the couple's communication may have deteriorated further, as was noted in other interactions between the two, to the point where many messages are misunderstood, not qualified, ignored, or not heard.

The second most frequently employed syndrome in the group was the "mind-reading" syndrome, often accompanied by what Watzlawick[14] refers to as the "spokesmanship" syndrome. In this case, spouse 1 claims he knows what the other is feeling or thinking. Without validating his assumptions, he explains to the rest of the group what his mate is feeling or thinking. He depends on his omnipotence and surprise to retain an advantage over the group and his spouse and to increase his self-esteem. This technique necessarily undercuts spouse 2's ability to speak for herself. In turn spouse 2 may resign herself and let spouse 1 continue to speak for her, may disagree for disagreement's sake, or may respond likewise, indicating she too is capable of reading minds, namely her mate's.

The following example illustrates how another couple, Pete and Esther, participated in both the mind-reading and spokesmanship syndromes.

PETE: (passively reclining in his chair, silent and seemingly uninvolved in the discussion)

NURSE: Pete, what are you thinking about?

PETE: Uh (grunts and nods head)

ESTHER: He's like this all the time . . . Pete doesn't love me; I don't know why he stays with me. (apparently making a statement and hoping to get feedback from Pete at the same time)

OTHERS:	(look surprised but do not challenge Esther's ability to speak for Pete)
PETE:	(silent, looking somewhat disgusted)
NURSE:	Did you hear what Esther said, Pete?
PETE:	Yes (begrudgingly)
NURSE:	It sounded to me as if she wanted to know if this was how you felt about her.
PETE:	She knows why I'm staying with her.

In this example of dialogue Esther suggests to the group that she knows what Pete is feeling in the group and how he feels about her without validating her assumptions. She gives a clue, however, that she does want feedback from Pete himself. The group is surprised by Esther's statements and her ability to speak for Pete; they do not challenge her ability to do so. Esther is portrayed as someone who "knows" and yet belittles herself by suggesting she is "unloved." What Esther may not realize is that her mind-reading and spokesmanship techniques undermine both her attempts to get feedback from Pete and Pete's ability to speak for himself. Pete seems on the one hand to resign himself to the fact that Esther is speaking for him but on the other hand seems to counter likewise by indicating he too can read minds; that is, he knows that Esther knows how he feels. Since he can read her mind, and she, his, there is no need for him to give her feedback.

Emergence and outcome of syndromes

The emergence and outcome of these dysfunctional communication syndromes in the group were seen to be indicative of total group functioning, as well as of individual member's anxiety. Syndromes appeared early in the formation of the group. This was believed to be caused by the members' generally high level of anxiety, and also the beginning stage was an appropriate time to rehearse histories that had caused couples to seek help. Wittingly or unwittingly, couples demonstrated those syndromes that had had a disruptive influence on their communication. These syndromes reappeared in the group periodically when individual or group anxiety was high with relationship to the process or content of the group. For example, when the nurse questioned the group's motivation to work on problems, members' anxiety rose and syndromes reappeared.

The outcome of these syndromes seemed to reflect a number of intrapersonal and interpersonal factors in the group. If the level of anxiety of a dysfunctional spouse was decreased by a change in the group's approach to him or by interventions of the nurse, these syndromes were often temporarily abandoned. If, however, group members identified with either of the dysfunctional pair and contributed to the dysfunctional dialogue, the syndrome was often perpetuated and tended to pervade total group interaction. In the following dialogue both Nadine and Esther indulge in the mind-reading syndrome:

ESTHER:	I didn't marry Pete out of love either . . . I know he didn't love me at the time. (pause) I don't know why he stays . . . I know he doesn't love me . . .
NADINE:	Yeah, I don't know why Joe doesn't get someone else, why he wants me back . . . I know he doesn't love me.

Nadine and Esther conclude that they have similar marital situations. Joe and Pete do not bother to contradict the fact that their wives have formulated correct evaluations of them.

The nurse's role

Although the nurse may unwittingly participate in continuing the use of syndromes in the group, he can be instrumental in discouraging the use of syndromes in the group. He can be helpful in aiding individual couples and the group to become aware of syndromes and of how they pervade interactions.

The following example of interaction from the group illustrates how the nurse might stop dialogue reminiscent of syndromes and comment on threats felt by a couple prior to the emergence of the syndrome in order that they understand what provokes their dysfunctional communication patterns.

ESTHER: I don't know what I'm going to do now.
NURSE: It would seem since Pete just got a steady job that you might feel more secure now; I don't understand.
ESTHER: I don't feel more secure.
PETE: (to Esther) What do you want from me, didn't I . . . and didn't I . . . ?
ESTHER: I know I'm not a good wife but *you* . . .
PETE: Don't I . . . ?
NURSE: Listen, . . . I think you both want to know that you are a good husband or wife— that you, Pete, are a good husband to Esther, and you, Esther, are a good wife to Pete.
ESTHER: (interrupts nurse) I don't think I'm a good wife.

The nurse attempted to stop the dialogue, which was reminiscent of variations of the blame syndrome, and to reflect on how both felt prior to the emergence of the syndrome, for example, that they both felt that their image of being an adequate or "good" husband or wife was being threatened. What the nurse may have done in addition was to comment about the threat felt and about how it was necessary for both to defend themselves.

The nurse could also comment about other members' parts in perpetuating syndromes or on how syndromes pervade the couple's interaction in the group and outside the group. The following dialogue is a continuation of Pete and Esther's interaction.

NURSE: Joe, how do you see Pete and Esther's situation?
JOE: Well—heh heh—(seemingly trying to be diplomatic) I think Esther doesn't want to be happy—to let herself feel happy.

At this time the nurse may have pointed out that Joe is implying the problem rests solely with Esther and may have suggested how this idea, although it could be a valid interpretation, would perpetuate the myth that problems are due to one mate's behavior and therefore necessitate change in only one spouse.

To encourage couples to experiment with more effective patterns of relating, the nurse merely gave positive reinforcement to new patterns by giving speical recognition to the change. The following is an example of dialogue between the nurse and Nadine. Nadine, as was pointed out in previous dialogue, utilizes the blame syndrome frequently.

NADINE: Well, I talked with the kids and I think Joe isn't the only problem . . . the kids have problems at school, I mean, there are some problems that don't have to do with Joe.

NURSE: Nadine, this is different for you. I notice that you are not blaming Joe for everything now.

NADINE: Yes . . . well, yes . . .

The nurse's ultimate aim was for Nadine to begin to acknowledge her part in the problematic relationship with Joe, to acknowledge that she, as well as Joe, has contributed to their problems, and that any change must involve both.

In summary, dysfunctional communication syndromes become integrated into systems of many couples' interaction. Their emergence in a group setting is indicative of total group functioning, as well as of individual member's anxiety. The nurse group leaders can employ various interventions that would be helpful in encouraging members to abandon these syndromes: (1) they can recognize and stop dialogue reminiscent of syndromes; (2) they can comment about the threat members feel just prior to the emergence of the syndrome; (3) they can comment on other members' parts in perpetuating these syndromes; (4) they can describe how these syndromes pervade the couples' interaction in the group and outside the group; and (5) they can encourage members to experiment with more effective patterns of relating.

Case study 2. Individual inclusion and group cohesion problems in multiple family group therapy*

Individual inclusion and group cohesion problems can plague most group therapy groups. These problems have been assessed on the basis of a number of characteristics of groups, for example, the degree of identification of members with the group, degree of groupness, degree of social isolation of members, and degree one feels he "fits" into the group and is included by others.

Group cohesion is seen here more generally as members' sense of belongingness, whereas needs for inclusion are referred to as needs around the question of "in or out." The need for inclusion, explains Schutz,[11] begins with the establishment of the group when people come face to face and decide how they are going to "fit" in the group. Anxiety around inclusion can give rise to individual-centered behavior, such as overtalking, extreme withdrawal, or recitation of other previous experiences.

The problems of unmet inclusion needs and lack of group cohesion come under examination here as I relate how coalition attempts in a multiple family therapy group serve as clues about what was concerning individual members and affecting the members' sense of belongingness in the group.

---

*Modified from Marram, G. D.: Coalition attempts in multiple family group therapy—indicators of individual inclusion and group cohesion problems, J. Psychiatr. Nurs. **10:**21-23, 1972.

Interventions pertinent to a nurse's role as cotherapist will be discussed in light of providing for inclusion needs of members and furthering group cohesiveness by acknowledging coalition premises: (1) problems of group cohesion and individual inclusion are not mutually exclusive, and (2) therapeutic change is influenced by the degree of the members' inclusion and by the degree of group cohesion. Inclusion of members is essential to formation of group cohesion or to a sense of belonging. When each member is informed about other members and sees himself and others as part of the group, cohesion is likely to develop. Likewise group cohesiveness enables members to establish themselves as specific individuals in the group. The therapeutic value of group cohesion has been acknowledged by many theorists.

I agree with Jerome Frank,[4] who explains that group cohesion can support self-esteem of members and thus increase members' tolerance for unpleasant emotions and their ability to function as responsible individuals. The degree to which members feel included influences their positive identification with the group and their commitment to the group's therapeutic goals.

The multiple family therapy group in which I served as nurse cotherapist was a heterogeneous group in an inpatient neuropsychiatric institute. Patients differed in age, sex, diagnoses, number of admissions to the hospital, and present length of stay. The number of patients attending the group meetings varied from meeting to meeting but was usually between four and six. Although some had as many as four members of their immediate family present, others had no family members present at group sessions. There was a constant turnover of auxiliary cotherapists, but two therapists attended regularly—the nurse cotherapist and a psychiatric resident. The group was essentially an ongoing group based on current hospital population. At the time I entered as cotherapist, one new member with his wife and another new member who had no family present had been added to the group. The other three patients and two families had spent approximately three sessions together. The goal for the group was explicitly stated by the psychiatric resident: "to discuss family concerns."

Coalition attempts were viewed here as two or more persons joined for the purpose of receiving support or consent from the other. This "sounding out" process is designed to create an ambiguous situation in which others are forced to respond by ignoring it, tactfully countering it, or by responding in a similarly ambiguous way. It is unusual enough behavior to get attention from others, yet not enough to be rejected. Coalition attempts over the period of two sessions enabled me to make a beginning assessment of problems in the group.

Selected examples of coalition attempts will be described here. It is important to note that while these attempts were made, the rest of the group were exhibiting behaviors that provided the therapists with additional clues about group problems with inclusion of members and with the members' sense of belongingness.

Example—Chuck and the group

Present at this session of the group, in addition to therapists 1 and 2 (the psychiatric resident and nurse cotherapist, respectively), were four patients: Joe, Cathi,

Chuck, and "the professor," five adult family members, and one other adolescent family member.

Joe and his two parents were talking about a specific family problem, occasionally directing questions to therapist 1 but virtually ignoring the rest of the group. Three adult family members appeared to be listening to the dialogue between Joe and his parents. Cathi, an adolescent patient, was fidgeting in her chair and swinging her legs, while her teenage sister sat sideways in her chair, turned away from the rest of the group. Another patient, Chuck, sat quietly in his chair next to therapist 2. As Joe asked therapist 1 what would help him get better and therapist 1 redirected the question to Joe, Chuck turned to therapist 2 and replied in a hushed voice, "He's trying to be evasive, isn't he?" Therapist 2 responded considerately, "Do you have something to contribute to the group, Chuck?" whereupon Chuck revealed that he wanted to tell the group about his problems but thought he could not talk because he did not have a family present.

Chuck's behavior was interpreted as an attempt to gain support from therapist 2 by turning to her instead of speaking to the group first. His attempt to get agreement on something that had transpired in the group indicated his desire for support of his opinions—as was implied, "Didn't therapist 2 agree?" He appeared to want consent not only to voice his opinion about what was happening in the group but also to be included in the group, where he felt he did not belong. The sounding out process was abnormal enough to draw attention but was countered and rechanneled in a way to ensure that Chuck would in fact be included and would be given the message that he was worthy of being included and in fact did belong. When his pattern of sending indirect messages was checked, he was enabled to verbalize his real concerns to the total group. Chuck's indirect and direct messages provided the therapists and the group as a whole with an opportunity to look at the possibility of some unmet inclusion needs and feelings of not belonging, as well as at problems of members drifting from the current discussions going on in the group.

Example—Cathi and the group

In the following session still other examples of coalition attempts appeared. At this session Chuck had begun to discuss his problems concerning drug addiction. His communication was flagged by loose associations and overloading others with too much information, but no one interrupted him to seek clarification.

Cathi began to giggle. She and her teenage sister sitting next to her appeared to be sharing a funny secret. Chuck continued to talk without verbally acknowledging the giggling. Therapist 2 asked Cathi whether she had something to contribute to the entire group. Cathi responded, "I don't understand what Chuck is talking about." Other members then asked Chuck to fill in missing parts of his story, indicating that more than one in the group was not comprehending him. Because members could not understand what Chuck was talking about, their mutual anxiety about being included was heightened. Cathi verbalized that she felt "out of it," and outside the group she indicated to therapist 2 that she did not understand what was being discussed and was afraid to ask for an explanation because "adults don't like to explain—I mean everyone *seemed* to understand, except me." Cathi's problems of feeling excluded and not bélonging were representative of problems that plagued the whole group.

That there might have been problems about inclusion of members and cohesiveness in this therapy group might have been concluded from the description of the group itself. The heterogeneity of the group, the continual turnover of members, and the assigned goal rigidly interpreted—to discuss family concerns—were factors influencing the group's ability to develop cohesion and provide for inclusion needs.

Intervening

When groups are obviously in beginning phases of development and inclusion is an issue, it is best to acknowledge coalitions as attempts to get support and clues that members may want to be brought into the group. An individual who seeks recognition, obscure as it may seem, may have an underlying wish to be brought into the group. Hidden communication must be acknowledged and clarified if inclusion of members in the group is to be achieved.

The cotherapist's role is not only one of observer but also one of expediter. He can encourage members to overcome feelings of anxiety and indecision and reservations about expressing themselves more directly in the group by acknowledging without criticism the members' attempts to be accepted into the group.

By acknowledging the group members' coalition attempts, the therapist can counter less constructive communication and reinforce more constructive patterns. By accepting the parts of Chuck's and Cathi's communication that were understood, these members were encouraged to clarify and verbalize their intended communication for the total group. Their indirect messages were thus replaced with more constructive patterns of verbalizing their intended messages.

As evidenced in this multiple family group, patients are initially unable to substitute their coalition attempts with more direct expressions, for example, Chuck's remark, "I don't feel like I can talk in this group because I don't have a family present." Thus it is the task of the therapists to help decipher any hidden messages by first acknowledging these attempts as actual messages to the group.

Finally, acknowledging coalitions gives the therapists a better understanding of additional factors influencing group cohesion and the members' inclusion in the group. These discussions exemplified such problems as members not feeling included because they did not understand what was being talked about or members feeling they did not belong because they did not have a family member present in the group. The therapist's clarification of communications and interpretation of the goals of the group increased the members' feelings of belongingness and inclusion in the group.

Acknowledging coalition attempts also stimulated the therapists to examine their own behavior and how they might be influencing members to feel that they must first gain support from others prior to talking to the total group. One therapist discovered that he might have been intentionally keeping some members from participating in the group because of his fear of losing control of the group. Group members may have been aware of his attempts to discourage their participation and consequently felt a need for additional support to bring their attempts into the group.

Acknowledging coalition attempts enables the therapist to (1) make room for members not included by recognizing attempts of those seeking inclusion, obscure as they may seem; (2) set examples for future more constructive communication by reinforcing constructive patterns and countering less constructive communication, and (3) detect additional factors influencing group cohesion and inclusion of members, which can then be manipulated to the advantage of the group and its members.

The nurse group therapist has a prominent part in directing a group toward development of group cohesion and providing for inclusion of members. Through the nurse's interventions the group members will be enabled to communicate and converse in an endeavor to achieve group cohesion.

Case study 3. Recurrent group focal conflict in the formative phase of group psychotherapy[*]

Nurse group therapists must speculate about latent content and covert forces operating within a group if meaningful therapeutic interventions are to be made. Likewise their response to covert forces will influence the nature of the patient's therapeutic experience in the group.

The group focal conflict theory as put forth by Whitaker and Liebermann[15] presents a systematized approach to viewing content and covert group forces. Whitaker and Liebermann[15] and Ezriel,[3] as well as many other group theorists, consider that covert group forces are potent elements in determining the nature of the patient's therapeutic experience and that the therapist who can utilize group forces properly can provide maximum benefits to the members of his group.

It is my purpose here not only to identify and describe a recurrent group focal conflict in the formative phase of a group therapy group but also to discuss the relevancy of certain interventions and conclusions on the part of the nurse group therapist in light of this particular theoretical framework.

The group therapy group described here consisted of six to eight men hospitalized on an acute treatment ward in a psychiatric institution. These patients differed in the severity of their illness and varied in diagnoses but included one psychopath, three paranoid types, and two with depressive reactions. All had had at least one former hospitalization experience.

The group focal conflict observed to be operant in beginning sessions of this therapy group revolved around the wish to be helped through revealing one's personal problems and the fear of attack, harm, and increased sickness through contact with other sick people. Group focal conflicts characteristically involve a wish or disturbing motive and a fear or reactive motive. Group focal conflict solutions that arise in response to both the disturbing and reactive motives are compromises between the opposing forces and may be either enabling or restrictive in nature. Solutions

[*]Modified from Marram, G. D.: Latent content and covert group forces in therapy with acute psychiatric patient, J. Psychiatr. Nurs. **9:**24-27, 1971.

are enabling if they are directed at alleviating fears and also at maximizing gratification of the disturbing motive. A restrictive solution does not allow for expression or satisfaction of the disturbing motive and is directed at alleviating fears.

The solutions that developed in early sessions of the therapy group discussed here were principally restrictive in that they allowed for little satisfaction or expression of the disturbing motive. These solutions constituted a culture in which patients' thoughts and feelings could not be constructively expressed and examined; members were largely restricted by the feared consequences of revealing personal problems and were faced with a limited range of behaviors to meet their needs for inclusion in the group—to be included and to include others.[11] These solutions were helpful in one sense, however, in that they alleviated initial anxiety of members in the group and made the group situation viable, allowing members to be included "on safe grounds" and the group to remain intact.

The following examples from the group will illustrate the presence of the recurrent group focal conflict—the wish to be helped through revealing one's personal problems and the fear of attack, harm, and increased sickness through contact with other sick people—and the solutions that were adopted, as well as the interventions by two nurse therapists, therapist 1 and therapist 2, which were relevant to the outcome of the conflict and the therapeutic experience of the patients.

Emergence of the conflict—reinforcing restrictive solutions

The following excerpt from the first session of the group illustrates the emergence of the disturbing and reactive motives and beginning restrictive solutions. Therapist 1 intervened by reinforcing a restrictive solution in order to avoid overwhelming anxiety in the group.

Members had revealed that they "really didn't have anything to say," and then focused the discussion on the therapists, seemingly to decrease their own anxiety. When one member had posed the norm: "group therapy is for talking about personal, psychological problems," anxiety increased, and another member, Mr. W., in response to his fear about talking in the group replied, "Well, it couldn't be confidential, it's in the group."

Another patient, Mr. R., apparently appreciative of the other's concern yet convinced the purpose of the group should be to talk about problems, responded (to Mr. W.), "You would like a little more privacy; well, it's a group meeting. You have something to express in regard to your personal problem—I really can't say. You'd better not express it here."

Mr. R.'s suggestion to avoid bringing up personal problems was in direct opposition to his desire to make the group a place where one could talk about "personal, psychological problems." A solution "not to express it here" evolved in light of members' fear of the consequences of exposing one's problems to the group. This solution alleviated members' fears at the expense of gratifying or expressing the disturbing motive.

Therapist 1 chose, rather than to oppose the restrictive solution suggested by Mr. R., "not to express it here," to allow for the temporary use of this solution.

Therapist 1: "I don't expect members to express personal problems if they are not ready. We are getting to know each other."

Whitaker and Liebermann[15] explain that sometimes the therapist will cooperate in maintaining a restrictive solution to avoid overwhelming anxiety in the group and that this stance is particularly important during the formative phase. Therapist 1 reinforced the restrictive solution to alleviate anxiety about the disturbing motive and at the same time lessened the threat of being excluded if one could not expose his problems to the group.

The following interchange suggests that, despite therapist 1's attempts at alleviating the reactive motive, fears predominated in the group. These fears were projected to the larger community and included the element of fear of being made sicker through contact with other sick people.

Mr. R.: "Mental illness could be created here . . . this might add to one's illness."

The therapists did not expose the fear as one existing in reference to the current group situation. Whitaker and Liebermann[15] warn the therapist not to capitalize too much on a current group focal conflict when patients may not be able to handle interpretations without extreme anxiety.

With the expression of these fears the remaining group conclusion was that one could not trust the group and therefore should not expose one's personal problems; the concurrent solution was to talk about such superficial topics as "Where are you from?" and "What are you going to do when you get out of the hospital?" These topics seemed not to be important in themselves but served as vehicles for members to get to know one another.

It is important to note that therapist 1's intervention that encouraged the restrictive solution may have served to increase some patients' fears of satisfying their desire to expose their problems, in that the therapist's hesitancy was further proof to them that gratifying their wish at this time was "dangerous" rather than "not appropriate for all."

Reemergence of the conflict—encouraging enabling solutions

The following session of the group illustrates the reemergence of the conflict. The therapists in this case encourage an enabling solution, which promotes reality testing by the members and partial satisfaction of the disturbing motive.

Doubt and suspicion about being able to trust group members and the therapists predominated in this session, along with a dim hope that one might be able to talk about his problems. Two patients were indicating that the important aspect of the reactive motive was the possiblity of being made sicker through contact with other sick people.

Mr. R.: "With them around . . . I mean, mental illness could be created here."

The reactive motive prevailed as patients discussed how one gets worse being in a mental institution and as they expressed fears of becoming impotent: "People will do things to you or make you do them; you are made to feel helpless, and your future is more determined by others than by your own mastery and control."

Patients began to synthesize their fears and project them onto an object, the therapists' tape recorder. The tape recorder was imputed with powers to do harm to members.

Mr. T.: "It's spooky" (referring to the tape recorder).

All laughed.

Mr. M. (to the therapists): "What do you use them for? I suppose you can use one for a lot of things, if you wanted to blackmail someone."

Therapist 1's spontaneous response aided in decreasing anxiety about the magical and harmful nature of the recorder and the therapists.

Therapist 1: "Be assured, Mr. B. (therapist 2) and I are not using it to blackmail you."

Mr. M. and Mr. R. laughed with recognition that such a statement would be reassuring to them.

Members then began to ask a number of questions about how the therapists were using problems brought out in the group. They wanted to know what happened to the tapes after meetings, who else heard the tapes, and what parts would be kept confidential. Members for the first time were beginning to test out real consequences of revealing their problems in the group, to compare the real with their fantasized dangers. The therapists encouraged the patients' checking out processes, thereby fostering an enabling solution. Patients realized that the consequences they feared had no real basis and that perhaps they could reveal their concerns. Whitaker and Liebermann,[15] Ezriel,[3] Johnson,[5] and others agree that reality testing in a group is essential to the individual's therapeutic experience and that reality testing can reduce taboos and fears and enable patients to have diminished feelings of isolation and a release of impounded feelings, as well as improved self-assertion.

Fears subsided in the group with the reassurance from the therapists that no harm would come to them if they revealed their personal problems in front of the tape recorder and the therapists. Members banned together to eliminate any further dangers by expressing that certainly everyone of them had problems; they were alike in this respect, and members should not criticize one another. What followed was a sporadic attempt to look at a number of members' concerns. Members expressed feelings they had about being treated like "babies" on the ward and about being pushed into jobs they did not like.

Reemergence of the conflict—proposing a restrictive solution inappropriately

In a later session the disturbing and reactive motives were expressed simultaneously by one patient who seemed to be impatient for an enabling solution whereby the disturbing motive could be more successfully gratified. Therapist 1, instead of capitalizing on the insight and motivation this patient brought to the group, suggested a restrictive solution, which temporarily closed off possibilities for more enabling solutions. Therapist 2 recognized the needless use of a restrictive solution and reinstated an enabling solution.

Mr. R.: "I see part of the problem here is to discuss personal problems; we are sitting now; no one is expressing his problems. . . ."

Other members agreed and said that they should get on with talking about "real" problems. Mr. R.'s implied directive "to get on with it" was an enabling solution in that it was directed toward relinquishing fears and allowing for some expression and satisfaction of the disturbing motive. Therapist 1, however, gauging the necessity of her intervention by her observations of nonverbal behavior, blocked this solution, thinking some patients were not ready to expose their problems to the group.

Therapist 1: "I think some of you might not be ready to talk about personal problems."

Therapist 1 operated on the assumption that some patients could not yet tolerate talking about their problems in the group without undue anxiety. Her response not only tended to block the enabling solution but also tended to disqualify Mr. R.'s attempts and exclude his contributions. Whitaker and Liebermann[15] warn that the therapist sometimes makes errors that prevent enabling solutions and that decrease safety for particular patients. What is viable for the therapist may oppose an enabling solution. The therapist in this case recognized that her own anxiety and preconceptions about members may have contributed to her cutting off Mr. R. and her utilizing unnecessary precautions.

Therapist 2 was able to reintroduce a more enabling solution.

Therapist 2: "What do others think about talking about personal problems?"

This intervention countered the restrictive solution and enabled patients to weigh again the possibility of talking about problems and allowing for further gratification of the disturbing motive. One member, Mr. R., understood therapist 2's comments as permission and the "go-ahead" and began to reveal his personal problem relating to his former suicide attempts. Having related part of his concern, he stopped.

Mr. R.: "I can't be the only one, everybody has to pitch in and talk together."

Therapist 1: "You mean if you talk about your problems you want everyone to share problems?"

Therapist 1's statement was geared toward reinforcing the norm that more than one member be expected to discuss his problems and toward clarifying Mr. R.'s concern.

Mr. R.: "Yeah, you know, find out what the other person's problems are; everybody should dig in, uh, help out one another that way."

Mr. R. seemed to be insuring himself against "being the only one" and against being criticized instead of helped by the others. The therapists continued to clarify with Mr. R. his fears of others' responses to his problems and asked if others had these concerns. One patient replied that he did not worry too much about what others said and began to ask Mr. R. about his suicide attempts. The discussion was expanded to include concerns about controlling unacceptable behavior in general, and drinking abuse specifically.

The reintroduction of an enabling solution here prevented members from resorting to a habitual, restrictive solution. Both therapists recognized the misuse of a restrictive solution and intervened to encourage further gratification of the disturbing motive and further checking out of fears.

In conclusion, I have identified and described a recurrent group focal conflict expressed during the formative phase of one group therapy group. Interventions by the two nurse group therapists were discussed in light of the focal conflict theoretical model. The nurses' responses to the group conflicts and the group solutions to the conflicts were seen to be instrumental in reinforcing necessary restrictive solutions and encouraging more enabling solutions, but also possibly encouraging restrictive solutions inappropriately. I maintain that covert forces such as those associated with group focal conflicts are important elements in determining members' experiences in a group. The nurse must speculate about the meaning and significance of these covert forces if meaningful interventions are to be made. As indicated in this case study the nurses' responses to these forces did influence the nature of the patients' therapeutic experiences in the group.

Case study 4. The impact of a sensitivity group on the self-esteem and self-concept of members of a profession*

In an increasingly complex and industrialized society two inevitable by-products are (1) the highly technical occupational roles it creates and (2) the consequences of a greater number of roles from which to choose. Highly technical and professional occupational roles, because of the time required in preparation for them and because of the continued dedication they enlist, demand priority over other roles. Individuals are necessarily faced with the problem of becoming dependent on their occupation as a source of satisfaction for various personal needs and as an avenue for increased self-growth, which cannot be met by a single role orientation. One alternative is to avoid looking at oneself in terms of one's professional role in order to discover all aspects of the self "as a whole person."

I examined the problems of role dependence and role detachment in two sensitivity groups of registered nurses. To measure the effect the sensitivity group experiences had on the members' role detachment, role dependence, and overall level of self-esteem, I utilized questionnaires and interviews as well as my long-term observations of the groups. I held individual interviews prior to, midway through, and at the end of the sessions; optional written reports from members were also collected at these times. In addition, global self-esteem tests and ten-item Guttam scales of self-esteem developed by Rosenberg[9] were altered to measure nurses' self-esteem in general, with reference to social and everyday life situations and in reference to their job situations. These scales were administered at the beginning and end of the sessions.

Characteristics of two different sensitivity groups

One group, which will be referred to here as group A, consisted of six to eight professional nurses who participated, with myself as leader, in T-group sessions over an 8-month period. The other group, group B, consisted of six to eight profes-

*Modified from Marram, G. D.: What is happening to nurses? Int. Nurs. Rev. **16:**320-328, 1969.

sional nurses participating, also with myself as leader, in T-group sessions over a 3- to 4-month period. It is important to specify how these groups differed with respect to characteristics of members, since a great deal of what happened in these groups will be based on a comparison of the two groups with respect to these features. Group A was composed of nurses ranging in age from 24 to 37 years, but most were over 35. Six of them were head nurses, two were assistant head nurses, and one was a senior staff nurse. Most of these nurses had had over 5 years (and up to 13 years) of work experience in hospital nursing. They reported that most of their friends were nurses and that they themselves lived alone. Few of them belonged to many outside groups, such as social or recreational groups.

Group B members differed significantly from group A members. These nurses ranged in age from 22 to 25 years. All were general duty staff nurses with from 18 months to 3½ years nursing experience. They reported that most of their friends were nonnurses and that they lived with persons who were not nurses. They explained that they belonged to a variety of outside groups, for example, bridge, art, and young adult forum groups.

The effects of T-group experience for these two groups seemed to have similar results, although in each group the problems were somewhat different. Both groups seemed to move members toward greater role adjustment and self-actualization and to increase members' self-esteem. For group B this meant that members could think of themselves more specifically as nurses fulfilling technical and demanding roles. For group A this meant that members could begin to relinquish their concept of themselves only with reference to their role as nurse.

Processes of acquiring increased self-esteem in the two T-groups

Although group A members demonstrated an initial need to respond to one another with respect to nursing role specifications, group B members demonstrated discomfort with being seen as "only a nurse."

Group A members exhibited low self-regard when they described themselves in social situations. They did not like being stripped of important role features such as responsibility, status, and the nursing care setting. They spoke of themselves as not being "beautiful" or "socially mature"—criteria they felt were used to measure people in social and everyday living situations. The leader attempted to support individuals in their experience of inadequacy and to help them check out with others in the group whether their perceptions of themselves were in line with how others actually saw them. Because the goal of the T-group—increased sensitivity to one another as persons—did not allow them to assume typical nursing roles, they were encouraged in the group to look at themselves increasingly as "unique" and "total" human beings. Members demonstrated some insight as to their need for dependence on their role, such as was evident in their understanding: " . . . we are talking like nurses . . . because it's more comfortable."

Beginning sessions with group B members reflected some basic insecurities in members, but these insecurities were almost diametrically opposite to those of the older, more experienced nurses in group A. Members in group B initially wanted to be seen "outside" the role of nurse and were comfortable if they were not stereo-typed in the nurse's role. Low self-regard and insecurity for these members seemed to result when they could not define themselves as unique individuals in the group. There was a generalized concern that others in the group see them as "well-round-ed" individuals. There was a rejection of the heritage of the "old" nurse and a strong emphasis on the "new" nurse who was, characteristically, a "well-rounded per-son . . . not just a nurse." Problems and insecurities were talked about and described as belonging to the job situation; they included such problems as communicating with patients and with other nurses who were authority persons and older and more experienced than themselves. As in group A, I attempted to give members support and to encourage them to check out with one another whether these incompetencies were seen by others. Members were in the position to observe each other in their professional nursing roles on the units they worked and could give important feed-back to one another about how they saw each other helping patients and getting along with their superiors.

It is interesting to point out here that presession interviews had led me to antici-pate the differences in these groups. Both groups indicated a certain resistance to the experience, but for very different reasons.

In presession interviews with members of group A, individuals demonstrated questionable confidence in themselves as unique persons to add something to the group and in how they might fit into such a group, as well as questionable confi-dence in the group's ability to teach them something since nursing problems were not to be the focus. Group B members, on the other hand, liked the idea of being part of a group that had to do with other than the direct nursing situation. A few warned that if it were just going to be about nursing problems, then they would not be interested. This warning was interpreted as an attempt to ensure an environ-ment where they would not be evaluated as nurses. Both groups tended to generalize areas they needed to work on, lacking clarity about what areas of interpersonal func-tioning in which they were weakest. They could not identify specific problems but responded to vague problem areas as if they incorporated a large part of the self. Members in group A listed "having to work on skills with people"; Group B, "com-munication problems at work."

As sessions progressed, both groups demonstrated a greater ease in, on the one hand, responding outside their professional nursing role and, on the other hand, responding in their role as nurse on their units. In group A, members demonstrated satisfaction with themselves as persons. Evidence of their wish to be recognized and accepted as unique individuals was apparent in their concern to let the "real me" show through, "to show my real feelings." Members indicated that they did not think it would be disastrous to let their "real" selves be known to others; they were no longer afraid that they would be rejected by others, either in the group or in situ-ations outside the group. Members spoke less about concerns with role detachment in social and everyday situations and remarked about the "progress" they were ex-periencing in coping with their feelings on the "outside" or in behaving differently toward others downtown or at social affairs.

Group B individuals demonstrated an increasing ease with reference to themselves as nurses. They reported an increasing ability to work out problems with associates at work and began to visualize their associates as "people" just like them. They indicated increased tolerance of individuals despite how long they had been in nursing, what program they came from—the "old" or "new," and their level of skill as a nurse.

It is important to note that at these times both groups attributed their corresponding ease in relating to the effects of the group. They, on occasion, purposely set up situations, group B in the work situation and group A at social affairs, so that they might try out what they thought they had learned in the group through discussion and role playing. What seemed to be operating was that recollection of what went on in the T-group sessions served as a kind of "conscience" for the member, continuing to encourage her to experiment with change.[1] The T-group as a source of positive identification became apparent for members in both groups.

Midsession and final session interviews with both groups indicated that alterations in self-perceptions and in attitudes toward the usefulness of the group had occurred. Tolerance of oneself was related to tolerance of others and to the ability to pinpoint one's own problems so that they seemed less overwhelming and more amenable to change. These changes in members were attributed to increased feedback exchange within the T-groups, which enabled members to visualize a more realistic picture of the self according to others and to realize that their problems were shared by others.

Members indicated by way of the optional written reports that feedback was most valuable. In cases where members did not get feedback, vague generalizations about the self and self-depreciatory feelings seemed to show up on their written reports.

Although the results of the global self-esteem tests indicated varying levels of self-esteem among members at the end of the groups' sessions, it was possible to draw some generalizations about the groups. As a whole, members' self-esteem in each group increased from the time the group had started. Group A members' increase in self-esteem was significant when they were asked to rate themselves compared to others "in social and everyday life situations. . . ." Group B members' increase in self-esteem was significant when they were asked to rate themselves compared to others "on the job. . . ."

In summary then it was apparent here that concurrent T-group sessions aided members in these two groups to cope with the problems of role dependence and role detachment, that is, to move toward role adjustment and further self-actualization in order to increase their self-esteem when they defined themselves in or out of their professional role as nurse. The T-group format utilized here resembled most sensitivity training groups in which individuals learn about the effects of their interpersonal interactions in the group. These T-group sessions seemed to be helpful to members because they (1) provided a different experience where nurses could evaluate themselves in and out of their occupational roles, (2) provided members the necessary feedback to alter negative perceptions of the self in or out of their role, and (3) served as a reference group where identification was positive and individuals were valued as unique persons and women occupying a professional role. The leader's or trainer's function was primarily that of an observer and facilitator—one not only of inviting examination of significant interactions but also of encouraging the sharing of common problems and attitudes toward the self and igniting feedback channels that would allow members to know how others viewed them in the group. As members participated in the sessions, they received feedback from others that negated felt suspicions about their being inadequate as nurses or in social and everyday life situations. They became more comfortable in relating as nurses and as unique individuals.

Case study 5. Facilitating self-disclosure in a psychotherapy group

Self-concealment is a major factor in emotional disturbance. It denies man's need for a community feeling and identification with his fellowman and allows him to undercommit himself, according to Pratt and Tooley,[8] thereby leading to failure in his contractual relations with society. Such contractual failure can be as severe as to limit one's tie to reality; or, according to Jourard, lead to a pathological state where energy to conceal adds to stress and dulls awareness of one's inner experience.[6] Transactions with others must be through a facade, making loneliness and depression the consequence.

Self-disclosure, the sharing of thoughts and feelings with others, on the other hand, not only ties individuals to the community of mankind but acts to bring the individual in closer contact with himself—taking responsibility for this self—and benefiting from the fact that sharing releases his personal burden. Self-disclosure is a necessary ingredient for mental health and a crucial variable in successful psychotherapy of individuals.

The following description of the barriers against self-disclosure and interventions taken in a group psychotherapy group illustrate how group leaders may confront resistances to and facilitate greater personal self-disclosure. First, however, it is necessary to lay the theoretical groundwork for what we mean by self-disclosure and its relationship to psychotherapy in a group.

Self-disclosure and psychotherapy

Self-disclosure occurs when one person voluntarily tells one other, or a group of others, things about himself that these others are unlikely to know or discover readily from other sources.

Jourard's[6] view of psychological illness (both psychosis and neurosis) is that a degree of self-alienation has occurred where the individual has lied about or repressed his true feelings, wishes, and here-and-now experience. The opportunity to tell another person one's hopes and fears, joys and sorrows, and plans for the future and memories of the past relieves loneliness. Through self-disclosure a person also comes to know himself and becomes able to introspect honestly. The act of verbally stating one's own experience to another, making oneself known to him, according to Jourard, permits one to get outside of oneself and see himself as he is. Self-disclosure is a necessary condition leading to self-acceptance. Failure to disclose at all makes it impossible to receive acceptance of oneself by others.

Two kinds of self-disclosure

Egan[2] contributed to our knowledge of self-disclosure by differentiating between two different forms of disclosure: demographic and personal self-disclosure.

Demographic self-disclosure is pseudo-self-disclosure. It is communication about events from the past rather than present experiences; it is factual material rather than personal claims about one's feelings and thoughts. It is generally presented in a way that involves minimal personal or interpersonal risk. Revealing one's place of residence, kind of job, and where one went to school would be examples of demographic self-disclosure.

Personal self-disclosure, on the other hand, is far more revealing of one's feelings, needs, and fantasies. It involves interpersonal and personal risk of sharing oneself and usually invites self-disclosure by others as well as empathic responses.

Because personal self-disclosure is necessary for interpersonal relationships and fosters psychological health, it is perhaps the primary goal of psychotherapy.

Therapists agree that for any form of psychotherapy to occur, a patient or client must reveal himself. Some of this disclosure occurs unwittingly—but every instance is important. Much of the therapist's behavior is directed toward establishing a relationship to increase personal as opposed to demographic self-disclosure.

Research by Truax and Carkhuff[12] has shown us that there is a strong correlation between personal self-disclosure and constructive personality change and social adjustment. Many clinicians have reported a positive correlation between personal self-disclosure and self-esteem. The greater the degree of personal self-disclosure by individuals, the higher the levels of self-esteem of these same people.

Resistances to self-disclosure in a group psychotherapy group

A particular group psychotherapy group that I co-led had as its aim to increase self-esteem of members through continuous interaction where members would be able to share experiences and learn they were not alone with their problems. The objectives of the group experience stated that through consecutive group sessions, members will—

1. Experience an increase in self-worth and self-esteem through identification with the group and awareness of their coping strengths
2. Experience an increased sense of identity, preferences, and awareness of choices and responsibilities
3. Realize that their problems are not exclusive to them
4. Learn from others in the group new ways of coping with problems
5. Alter expectations of self and group along realistic criteria
6. Experience release of frustration and hopelessness within a supportive group atmosphere

The group formed an integral therapeutic effort for patients in an outpatient affective-disorder clinic. Members were either discharged inpatients or clients with no recent history of hospitalization. All members were diagnosed as having a minor or major affective disorder—bipolar or unipolar manic-depressive illness with a probable endogenous base. The group consisted of ten members, five men and five women, ranging in age from 30 to 47 years.

Personal self-disclosure to these members was a risk for many reasons. Yalom[16] identified some basic variables determining intensity of risk:

1. The nature of the disclosed material, for example, first-time disclosures carry more risk than material disclosed several times previously.
2. The probability that the receiver(s) will receive the disclosures as intended; for example, risk is lessened if the receiver understands, is sensitive to, and has experienced similar feelings or thoughts.
3. The probability that the receiver will reciprocate as the sender hoped he would, for example, would indicate his own vulnerability so that the person originally self-disclosing would not feel "out in the cold."

Each of these variables was important in this group of affective-disorder patients, making self-disclosure difficult for members and the role of the group leader an extremely challenging one.

Threats around disclosing will be identified specifically as (1) fear of revealing unacceptable thoughts and actions in the recent past or present (overbearing harsh superego judgements), (2) over concern with reactions of members and leaders, for example, fear of rejection, and (3) long-term use of denial and blocking to avoid painful realizations about self.

Depressive clients are notorious for their low self-esteem, harsh superego, and their destructive tendency to take anger and turn it inward against the self. Guilt, shame, and self-punishment characterize the judgments and behaviors of these individuals, making others' attempts to convince them of their self-worth often fruitless. Members can ward off a therapist's efforts by claiming the leader "doesn't really know the extent of my sins," "can't really help me," or "is not strong enough to confront my destructive impulses." It is the client's own sense of helplessness and hopelessness, together with his disbelief that he can or should be helped, that make this group experience with affective-disorder patients so challenging to the leaders.

Table 2 illustrates how the group changed in self-disclosure behavior as perceived by the leaders. Each leader independently rated the group after each session as to how self-disclosing members were; this table illustrates group patterns within the first fourteen group sessions. The leaders were to judge whether and to what degree members were self-disclosing. Table 2 also indicates two important drops in the extent to which members were self-disclosing following a period of gradual increase in self-disclosing communication. The first drop-off came after the addition of two new members; the second, after "too much" was disclosed by one member, making self-disclosure temporarily risky.

To participate in some level of personal self-disclosure, members must have faith that it is a useful objective and that it will be received kindly by others. Potent barriers to self-disclosure in the group were clearly members' fears of revealing un-

Table 2. Pattern of self-disclosure in sequential group sessions

Degree of personal self-disclosure	Session													
	1	2	3	4	5	6	7	8	9	10	11	12	13	14
Yes, very high							x		x					
Yes, moderately high			x		x	x		x		x		x	x	x
No, only slightly self-disclosing				x‡				x§			x‖			
Not at all self-disclosing		x†												
Unable to determine														
Varied greatly depending on member	x*													

* Varied from very to only slightly self-disclosing.
† Two members rated moderately self-disclosing.
‡ One member rated very high; another, moderately.
§ Two new members were added to the group.
‖ Sessions 11 and 12 followed a meeting of high self-disclosure when members were concerned about revealing too much.

acceptable thoughts, feelings, and actions, concerns one would be rejected by the group, and long-term use of denial as a defense mechanism.

In the beginning of the group the major kinds of self-disclosure were demographic; members related with some comfort their situational circumstances—why they were coming to the clinic, what medications they were taking, and what their symptoms had been in the past. They avoided disclosure of here-and-now problems they were having with family members or on the job or their doubts that they could help themselves. They viewed others' disclosure statements as if they were "spectators," without committing themselves to helping the sender make himself better understood.

One patient, Mrs. M., was telling the group she had just been discharged from the hospital:

MRS. S.: "Do you have any friends or family here?" (asking for factual information)
MRS. M.: "Yes, my husband . . . but we are separated; I'm living alone." (answering and giving hints she may have problems)
MRS. S.: "Oh—well—that's good—it helps to have somebody to turn to." (looks at the facts, not the circumstances that would lead to loneliness and fear)

Avoiding discussion of personal problems with loneliness, the group turned to a more superficial discussion of common symptoms and who was taking which medications. Empathy was feigned, if not lacking entirely; members tended to depersonalize their experiences despite leader attempts to counteract these defenses with statements such as—

L_1: "I wonder if you can tell us something about your problems." (refocus members on relevant problem issues)
L_2: "I'm trying to understand more about that episode—can you tell me specifically how you started the hassle? (asking member to elaborate on a problem)

A typical form of resistance was to block off further exploration.

MRS. S.: "I got so bad I had to have shock treatments. I don't remember now."

L₂: "It must have been hard for you feeling that "down." (confronting resistance by supporting patient in her experience of pain on recall)

MRS. S.: "I can't talk anymore about my problems." (resisting connecting feelings and experiences by blocking and maintaining that these experiences are a part of the unretrievable past)

It was clear to the leaders that safety to the group meant to stay away from self-disclosure that would elicit painful memories; demographic data that had been revealed several times in other interactions was "okay" because it allowed the group to block recall of meaningful, albeit painful, experiences.

Also, members could successfully ensure superficiality if they responded to others' attempts at self-disclosure with a passive, detached demeanor similar to that of spectators hearing and seeing something they could never truly feel themselves.

Feeling "okay" to reveal anything in depth at this point was restricted by anticipated pain in doing so, reexperiencing pain from the past and being expected to follow suit when allowing another to seek empathy and support through the same process.

Unacceptable thoughts and actions served as an intermittent barrier to self-disclosure with two members in particular. Examples of leader interventions in these cases highlight further complexities in facilitating self-disclosure.

With both Mrs. M. and Mr. F., chronic use of denial and blocking served to protect them, and in the case of Mrs. M. was a self-destructive outcome. Both Mr. F. and Mrs. M., in two separate group sessions, clearly had unacceptable thoughts and actions they were concealing from the group that contributed to their personal stress and loneliness.

Mr. F. remained silent in the group, fidgeting more than usual when other members talked about their problems. The stress of concealment that Jourard describes was clearly apparent. Leader 2, who was seeing him in individual therapy as well, could predict what personal events were preoccupying him. He had recently been drunk, harassed his wife and children from whom he was separated, and was rejected. His lawyer had warned him that his behavior would have to stop or he would be put in jail and would lose all visitation rights. He was extremely depressed and ashamed of his own behavior but could not use the group to ventilate or give him support.

L₁: "Mr. F., how are you tonight?" (acknowledging patient and asking for clarification)

MR. F.: "I'm okay." (denial)

L₁: "You don't look okay; I don't think you have to say that if you don't really feel it." (confronting patient with the conflicting verbal and nonverbal messages he was giving and at same time supporting patient to face where he really was)

Mr. F. opened up to reveal to the group what he had done, avoiding the reprimand incident with his lawyer but obviously ventilating, for him, some important facts about which he was ashamed. He recounted for the group how he had become upset thinking of his wife divorcing him and how she turned him away. He got drunk and protested outside her apartment door, creating a disturbance and upsetting his children. After revealing his story, Mr. F. relaxed and could better listen to others talk about their problems. In recounting the events, he was able to gain further insight into his feelings and why he took the actions he did.

Like Mr. F., Mrs. M. was resistant to bringing up the personal issues that were most important for her at the time. She was sympathetic and supportive to others who would share personal troubles. But in doing so it was possible for her to avoid revealing her own circumstances in the group. Again, leader 2 had knowledge through her one-to-one session with Mrs. M. that she was not sharing vital information with the group. Mrs. M. had revealed in her one-to-one session that she felt like committing suicide, that if her husband wanted a divorce and did not want to see her again, there was "no use in living." Mrs. M. appeared withdrawn and depressed in the group.

L₁: "Mrs. M., you look really different tonight; what is going on with you?" (opening up discussion of problems by acknowledging change in patient)

MRS. M.: "Well I'm feeling down I guess. Things are not going so well with my husband; he is more cold and aloof." (stays for a second on self before focusing on husband's behavior)

MRS. J.: "How do *you* feel about him?" (other patient reacts to Mrs. M. responding like a "victim")

MRS. M.: "Well, it would be a cop-out if I didn't look at my part."

L₂: "What would be a cop-out?" (looks directly at Mrs. M., confronting her with the expectation that her cop-out may be that she was not telling the group everything they needed to know about her)

MRS. M.: "Yes . . . well, I'm really depressed; if he doesn't want me, then I don't see any point to it. Our other therapist (who sees them for couple therapy) says we have a pattern where my husband has to save me; and I might be living out his suicidal wishes."

Mrs. M. continues on about her desperation and gets reinforcement from leader 2 for trusting the group enough to begin revealing her fantasies and fears to the group. Near the end of the session:

L₂: "Mrs. M., you shared some important things about yourself. I think it was important that you do this, let the group know what was going on with you." (acknowledging change in Mrs. M. and reinforcing the behavior change)

Encouraging self-disclosure in the group was not an easy task. The leaders utilized a variety of techniques to carefully move members toward greater personal self-disclosure. Refocusing patients on problem issues, acknowledging discrepancies in nonverbal and verbal behavior, acknowledging changes in patients from one session to another, confronting patients with their denial, and rewarding personal self-disclosure statements were interventions that, when timed appropriately, led to greater disclosure.

Another intervention, while it was used less frequently and is controversial, was that of leaders promoting self-disclosure by offering their own personal experiences. This technique was used with Mr. R., whose blocking of feelings was fortified by the fact that he claimed he had no models that believed "feelings" were "good" or useful.

Group discussion was focused on frustration and anger. Mr. R. had been explaining how his parents had never shown emotions of any kind and how he did not feel extremes of positive or negative feelings. Sharing how you felt was neither "manly" nor commonplace. He explained that consequently the women he had been in love with claimed he was not involved enough.

Leader 1 used an example of how he had been recently frustrated and how he felt like hitting and breaking something but did not. Mr. R. listened intently to the leaders' description of how he (the leader) was angry and felt like breaking the object of his frustrations. The leader was demonstrating two essential points: (1) it is okay to feel strong feelings and (2) to admit them to others (being that the leader was also male, the leader was role modeling an authority figure, which Mr. R. could emulate without confusion as to his sexual identity and manhood). This intervention had the effect of causing members to challenge Mr. R. to identify the feelings he "must have" and expect him to learn to be empathetic to them. The effect on Mr. R. was that he began to question his own responses and examine what was behind his reactions.

For example, when Mr. R. changed the subject in the group as another patient spoke of a painful experience, he was challenged:

L₁: "Mr. R., when Mrs. M. said that, you looked up at the ceiling and changed the subject as if you didn't feel anything."

MR. R.: (smiling uncomfortably) "Yes." (contemplating the reasons why he was uncomfortable)

At the next group meeting Mr. R. wondered about his depression and what his "lows" were really like: Would he change naturally? How depressed would he get? Mr. R. began to examine more intently his feelings and reactions as if he were a young child learning about life and himself for the first time.

The intervention where the leader uses personal self-disclosure to promote patient self-disclosure is a controversial one. In this instance it was important that some members have disclosure modeled for them so that they might more easily transcend their own resistances to expressing feelings, thoughts, and fantasies. From my point of view, leaders should have a specific rationale before employing this technique. There is always the possibility that the leader's intent will be misunderstood or that the leader, in revealing personal details, becomes concerned about whether he has revealed too much or stepped out of his professional role. Whereas this did not occur, the use of leader self-disclosure as an intervention should be well thought out before it is used.

In conclusion, personal self-disclosure is an essential ingredient in psychotherapy of any kind. The success of this group in meeting the objectives set forth depended on members being able to share personal feelings, fantasies, and painful events they had experienced. Disclosure was difficult to facilitate, however, with patients whose own self-judgments were often more harsh than that of the group and who used denial to reduce the pain of self-judgment. Direct confrontation, role modeling, and acknowledging metacommunication were most useful to the leaders in breaking through the barriers of self-concealment of these affective-disorder patients.

Case study 6. The problem of mutual withdrawal in an inpatient group milieu*

It is often the case that nurses think of their role as a group leader or group therapist only in the context of a formal group setting. Whereas the dynamics of group interaction are perhaps most clear-cut when we look at them within the confines of an enclosed small group, it is misleading to think of the nurse's role in such narrow terms. This case study deals intentionally with the nurse as a leader in a vaguely defined group atmosphere—a hospital milieu. Essentially we will look at the problems of member isolation—its underlying basis and how the nurse could effect change in the group milieu to decrease the phenomenon of mutual withdrawal between individuals in the milieu. This group does not consist solely of selected patients in an in-patient treatment unit, but contains staff members as well. The theory that will be used to explain the phenomenon will be the interpersonal and social-psychological foundations of Tudor[13] and Menzies.[7]

Nursing owes much to Tudor and her study, "A Sociopsychiatric Nursing Approach to Intervention in a Problem of Mutual Withdrawal on a Mental Hospital Ward." Tudor recognized the importance of the social context within which the patient resides, namely the ward setting. The characteristic attitudes and activities that constitute the staff's formal and informal participation are an integral part of the patient's living and will either move him toward health or away from it. Three general assumptions behind Tudor's pursuit were that the mode of participation or the patient's mental illness can be altered and influenced by the activities others direct toward him and, most important, that the patient's participation can change if the staff is aware of (1) the nature of the interpersonal situation it engages in with the patient and (2) the nature of the social arena within which their interpersonal exchanges take place. Tudor stresses the significance of the total social group context in affecting a variety of interpersonal relationships in regard to the patient, recognizes what is important in altering the social participation of the patient, and suggests methods by which the staff may be motivated to approach a heretofore isolated patient.

Of equal significance here is the theory of Menzies, which explains what factors motivate staff members to avoid patients. Menzies contributed to our understanding in this area by exploring various anxieties and the defense mechanisms utilized by the nursing staff toward patients in a general hospital. According to Menzies the

---

*Modified from Marram, G. D.: Toward a greater understanding of mutual withdrawal in a psychiatric setting, J. Psychiatr. Nurs. **7:**160-163, 1969.

sources of anxiety that necessitate some means of avoidance or withdrawal include the following:

1. Contact with illness and death
2. Unclear prognosis for the patient
3. Distasteful, frightening tasks
4. Strong and mixed feelings toward patients, such as guilt and anxiety

The defensive mechanisms against these sources are many but may include the following:

1. Simply terminating the nurse-patient relationship
2. Depersonalization or categorization of persons
3. Ritualistic performance of tasks

One can see the advantage of combining both Menzies' observations of sources of anxiety and possible defensive measures and Tudor's framework for viewing mutual withdrawal in interpreting a case of mutual withdrawal in a group of staff and patients in an inpatient psychiatric setting.

The isolated member

Mrs. K. was the isolated member of a group of patients and staff on a psychiatric unit. She was diagnosed as a "chronic paranoid schizophrenic" with a well-developed conclusive and logical delusional pattern. There were no marked effects on her intellectual processes, however. She was a 72-year-old grandmother, separated from her husband for more than 40 years. The death of her only child 3 years ago was believed to be an extremely stressful event in her life.

Mrs. K. protested that the Communist Party "railroaded" her into the hospital to prevent her from exposing evidence she had against them and that the hospital from which she was referred had verified that nothing was wrong with her. Mrs. K. also believed she had no need of therapeutic treatment and that she was confined in the hospital because of her efforts focused on "getting letters to the outside"—letters alleging the hospital to be operated by members of the "goon squad for the Communist Party" and charging other state officials with being connected with the Communists.

Mrs. K. evidenced a pattern of withdrawal on the unit. She remained within the confines of her room, not wishing to be identified as a patient. She did not attend formal group therapy sessions nor community meetings. She limited herself to reading books, working crossword puzzles, and writing letters—participating only in solitary activities. She avoided contacts with other patients because "It doesn't do them any good to see what they are doing to me here." Contact with the psychiatrist in charge of the unit caused her to become enraged: "Dr. R. has all the attributes of a dedicated Communist!" Contact with visiting doctors also angered her: "He is in cahoots with Dr. R." She stated that Dr. R. would not dare to come to talk with her and never speaks to her because she had told him, "I never want to speak to you again," and the visiting doctor had not returned because, "I got him interested in the Communist Party and he was going to look into it."

My relationship with Mrs. K. was basically oriented toward establishing a thera-peutic nurse-patient relationship based on mutual trust and acceptance whereby I was to encourage the more healthy aspects of Mrs. K.'s behavior. What arose from 'his relationship and from my contact with staff members, however, was a more general group leader role in which I attempted to alter the total group milieu in order to minimize this patient's isolation.

The staff and their relationship to the isolated member

Evidence of the staff members' avoidance-withdrawal was evident from Mrs. K.'s explanations that she was left alone and from observations of (1) an overall feeling of "helplessness" and active avoidance of direct contact with Mrs. K., (2) an attitude of dismissal toward Mrs. K., since she did not conform to the hospital routine and treatment regimen, and (3) some staff members' lack of information regarding Mrs. K. other than data gathered indirectly from brief contacts others had had with her. When staff members were asked, "What do you think of Mrs. K.?" it became evident that she aroused strong and mixed feelings in them such as anxiety, guilt, fear, and anger. The staff's defensive measures (outlined by Menzies) most com-monly employed to abate uncomfortable feelings about Mrs. K. but which furthered the avoidance-withdrawal pattern were (1) reduction of the impact of responsibility by delegation of it to superiors, (2) severing of the nurse-patient relationship, (3) depersonalization, categorization, and denial of the significance of the individual, (4) detachment and denial of feelings, (5) ritual performance of tasks, and (6) avoidance of change in attitude or behavior toward the patient.

The ward secretary explained that nothing was being done for Mrs. K. and that "she refused to go to any of the meetings." The staff members relieved their guilt feelings about shirking responsibility here by projecting the blame on the patient. The secretary's irritation at Mrs. K. for not conforming to the therapeutic regimen was evident, the finality of her response implying that change in attitude or approach to the patient was not forthcoming.

Reduction of the impact of responsibility was evident in the action of a new staff nurse who delegated responsibility for treatment decisions to others or superiors, saying she did not know what could be done for Mrs. K. but if Dr. S. were asked maybe he could suggest something. This nurse then wanted me to relate any further findings back to her, indicating that she had attempted to form a relationship with Mrs. K. but that the relationship had been severed. She had previously listened to Mrs. K. but challenged her delusional thoughts; and now, "I don't challenge her any more, she just gets more upset . . . I don't even try any more." Feelings of helplessness on the part of the nurse seemed to account in part for the early termina-tion of this nurse-patient relationship.

Both of Mrs. K.'s psychiatrists tended to categorize Mrs. K., depersonalizing their viewpoint and denying her significance as an individual: "She is a paranoid schizo-phrenic with a complex delusional system." Behind this depersonalizing approach to viewing Mrs. K. was some evidence of feelings of anxiety and doubt about their own behavior in her treatment. Although not admitting any difficulties in establishing a relationship with Mrs. K., one doctor responded hesitantly, "Have you been able to talk with her?" Another doctor had little first-hand information about Mrs. K., stating, "I've heard stories about her . . . but I've never talked to her."

An aide who had more direct contact with Mrs. K. indicated the conditional basis on which she related to Mrs. K., explaining that she does talk to Mrs. K. occasionally about "daily things" but never "goes in there (to Mrs. K.'s room) just to sit and talk." This aide stated that the staff members left Mrs. K. alone in her room at times when Mrs. K. would cry and get enraged and that "she likes to be alone in her room then." In talking about the patient's delusion the aide stated " . . . of course we can't believe her." There seemed to be several possible sources of anxiety and defensive measures here. The aide felt more comfortable in performing ritual tasks such as talking about "daily things" with Mrs. K. Fear of Mrs. K. and her expressions of emotion, as well as doubt about whether one might begin to believe the patient's delusional thoughts, may have been sources of anxiety.

The idea that Mrs. K. presented an out-and-out threat was evident in both the reports of another staff nurse and the ward social worker. The staff nurse explained that Mrs. K. "gives us trouble . . . " and that the chief psychiatrist of the hospital "tells us we must keep her locked up . . . ; when she accuses us of this you feel guilty because we *are actually keeping* her in here." Mrs. K. is a threat not only because she writes threatening letters but also because she arouses guilt feelings in staff members. The social worker warned me, "Oh . . . you'd better not associate with us. . . . You'll get like all the rest of us," meaning that Mrs. K. assumed the entire staff was connected in some way with the Communist Party.

Mrs. K. seemed to instill a mixture of strong feelings of guilt, fear, anxiety, and anger in the staff members. Most staff members seemed to be doubtful of ever succeeding in helping this patient or of knowing how to handle her. Others dismissed her by blaming Mrs. K. herself for these failures. Still others seemed more concerned with what threats Mrs. K. posed for them personally. The staff members tended to "leave her alone" and to rationalize their avoidance of her.

Even I was not immune to acquiring some of these same feelings and employing defensive measures to characteristically avoid Mrs. K. For example, pessimism about Mrs. K.'s prognosis, as well as identification with the psychological stress of withdrawal from the patient experienced by others, was anxiety-producing for me. At one point I found myself so overly dedicated in talking with the staff personnel to encourage them to interact with Mrs. K. that I had become tardy for a designated appointment with the patient. In one sense this measure was in fact a forfeiting of responsibility to others, which at the same time withdrew attention from the patient.

Mrs. K. responded to the staff's avoidance of her by remaining secluded, explaining "They treat me like a hotel guest. . . . They know they can't do anything to me."

The characteristic social process of interacting perpetuated by the attitude and behavior of both staff members and patient was not moving the patient toward health. Mrs. K. organized observations of how she was treated so that it might logically fit with her well-developed delusion, and she responded accordingly—as if in fact she were a hotel guest and did not have anything in common with the other patients. She would only seek out staff members when her "room and board" did not satisfy her. The staff in turn felt both helpless and responsible in some ways for allowing perpetuation of the myth this patient had designed.

The consequences of isolation of the mentally ill are well known to most therapists; with social isolation there is continued reliance on autistic inventions. For each staff member there were specific sources of anxiety that had led to utilization of various defensive measures against feelings of anxiety, guilt, fear, and anger —all of which resulted in avoidance-withdrawal behavior.

To combat a pattern of mutual withdrawal in this setting, I visualized goals to alter the social context. I did this by (1) instilling curiosity and interest about the patient in staff members, (2) communicating any successfully used methods of approach, and (3) aiding the staff in recognizing the complexities of their behavior and attitudes, particularly anxiety-producing stimuli and concurrent defensive measures they were employing, which not only caused them to avoid and withdraw from the patient but which also tended to perpetuate the pattern of mutual withdrawal. I felt that my own discussions of personal reactions and feelings about Mrs. K. would ease the staff's acceptance of similar feelings and reactions of their own without their consequently feeling more guilty about their behavior. I believed that the specialized attention given to staff members about their personal reactions to Mrs. K. would instill curiosity and interest and encourage them to try out new approaches with this patient. I was also cognizant of the importance of directing Mrs. K.'s interests and abilities to include relationships with those other than myself. To focus the patient's relationships to include others seemed to necessitate (1) enforcing basic trust in the patient of both herself and of others, (2) enforcing the patient's acceptance of herself and others, and (3) enforcing the patient's self-esteem, all of which might increase her interest in seeking out other relationships with both staff members and patients.

I maintain that an understanding of the phenomenon of mutual withdrawal, whether it is in a formal group setting or a more loosely defined group milieu, necessitates a dual perspective: consideration of Tudor's findings of the total social context in affecting a variety of interpersonal relationships and of Menzies' study of specific sources of anxiety and defense mechanisms that characterize the staff's relationship with a particular patient. To understand the nature of avoidance-withdrawal on the part of staff members, it is necessary to consider the specific sources of anxiety perceived within each individual's context of anxiety-producing situations and the specific repertoire of defenses available to the individual. The clinical case of Mrs. K. was cited as an example of the complexity of the breakdown of therapeutic contact and of the complex problem of mutual withdrawal in a psychiatric setting.

REFERENCES

1. Bennis, W. G., et al., editors: The planning of change, New York, 1961, Holt, Rinehart & Winston, p. 724.
2. Egan, G.: Encounter: group processes for interpersonal growth, Belmont, Calif., 1970, Brooks/Cole Publishing Co.

3. Ezriel, H.: A psychoanalytic approach to group treatment, Br. J. Med. Psychol. **23:**59-74, 1950.
4. Frank, J. D.: Group therapy in the mental hospital, Washington, D.C., 1955, American Psychiatric Association, Mental Hospital Service, p. 5.
5. Johnson, J. A.: Group therapy—a practical approach, New York, 1963, McGraw-Hill Book Co.
6. Jourard, S.: Healthy personality, New York, 1974, The Macmillan Co.
7. Menzies, I. E. P.: A case study in the functioning of social systems as a defense against anxiety: a report on a study on the nursing service of a general hospital, Hum. Rel. **13:** 95-121, 1960.
8. Pratt, S., and Tooley, J.: Human actualization teams: the perspective of contract psychology, Am. J. Orthopsychiatry **66:**881-895, 1966.
9. Rosenberg, M.: Society and the adolescent self-image, Princeton, N.J., 1965, Princeton University Press.
10. Satir, V.: Conjoint family therapy, Palo Alto, Calif., 1964, Science and Behavior Books.
11. Schutz, W. C.: FIRO: a 3-dimensional theory of interpersonal behavior, New York, 1958, Rinehart & Co., p. 14.
12. Truax, C., and Carkhuff, R.: Client and therapist transparency in the psychotherapist's encounter, J. Couns. Psychol. **14:**3-9, 1965.
13. Tudor, G. E.: A sociopsychiatric nursing approach to intervention in a problem of mutual withdrawal on a mental hospital ward, Psychiatry **15**(2):193-217, 1952.
14. Watzlawick, P.: An anthology of human communication, Palo Alto, Calif., 1964, Science and Behavior Books.
15. Whitaker, D. S., and Liebermann, M. A.: Psychotherapy through the group process, New York, 1964, Atherton Press.
16. Yalom, I.: The theory and practice of group psychotherapy, New York, 1970, Basic Books, Inc., Publishers.

SUGGESTED READINGS

Case study 1. Dysfunctional communication syndromes in a married couples group

Lederer, W. J., and Jackson, D. D.: The mirages of marriage, New York, 1968, W. W. Norton & Co.

Case study 2. Individual inclusion and group cohesion problems in multiple family group therapy

Benne, K., and Muntzan, B.: Human relations in curriculum change, New York, 1951, Dryden Press, p. 106.

Case study 3. Recurrent group focal conflict in the formative phase of group psychotherapy

Schutz, W. C.: The interpersonal underworld. In Schutz, W. C.: FIRO: a 3-dimensional theory of interpersonal behavior, New York, 1958, Rinehart & Co.

Case study 4. The impact of sensitivity groups on the self-esteem and self-concept of members of a profession

Adelson, D.: Self-valuation, social valuation, and self identity: a framework for social psychiatric inquiry, paper presented at International Congress of Social Psychiatry, London, 1964.
Burke, R. L., and Bennis, W. G.: Changes in perception of self and others during human relations training, Hum. Rel. **14:**165, 1961.
Davis, F., editor: The nursing profession, New York, 1966, John Wiley & Sons.
DeLevita, D. J.: The concept of identity, Paris, 1965, Mouton & Co.

Dittes, J. E.: Attractiveness of a group as a function of self-esteem and acceptance by the group, J. Abnorm. Psychol. **59:**77-82, 1959.

Sherif, M.: The self and reference groups—meeting ground of individual and group approaches, Ann. N.Y. Acad. Sci. **96:**797-813, 1962.

Sherwood, J.: Self identity and referent others, Sociometry **28:**66-81, 1965.

Shibutani, T.: Society and personality—an interaction approach, Englewood Cliffs, N.J., 1961, Prentice-Hall.

Taves, M. J., et al.: Role conception and vocational success and satisfaction: a study of student and professional nurses, Columbus, Ohio, 1963, Ohio State University Bureau of Business Research.

Zander, A., et al.: Unity of group, identification with group and self-esteem of members, J. Pers. **28:**463, 1960.

Case study 5. Facilitating self-disclosure in a psychotherapy group

Cozby, P.: Self-disclosure: a literature review, Psychol. Bull. **79:**73-91, 1973.

Jourard, S.: Self-disclosure: an experimental analysis of the transparent self, New York, 1971, John Wiley & Sons.

Pearce, W., and Sharp, S.: Self-disclosing communication, J. Commun. **23:**409-425, 1973.

Wenburg, J., and Wilmont, W.: The personal communication process, New York, 1973, John Wiley & Sons.

Yalom, I.: The theory and practice of group psychotherapy, New York, 1976, Basic Books, Inc., Publishers.

Case study 6. The problem of mutual withdrawal in an inpatient group milieu

Stanton, A., and Schwartz, M.: The mental hospital, New York, 1954, Basic Books, Inc., Publishers.

EXERCISE FOR PART THREE: ANALYZING A CASE STUDY

The purpose of this exercise is to give the reader an opportunity to employ the discussion of leadership functions and interventions in Chapter 8 and of case studies in Chapter 10 through analyzing an actual group experience from the leadership perspective. The reader is encouraged to examine the dialogue of a case study below and consider the following questions: (1) What problems do you perceive with reference to the group as a whole and with reference to individuals in the group? (2) What did the nurse group leader do and what would you have done? (3) What theoretical bases—principles and concepts—would you use to support your functions and interventions in the group?

Case study

This is a group of five or six terminally ill cancer patients and their spouses meeting for the first time with the nurse group leader in a solarium of a general hospital unit. The patients are hospitalized to undergo radiation and chemotherapy. The nurse plans to meet with this group twice a week in the evenings from 7:30 to 8:30 in order to help members and family discuss openly and share with others the frightening aspects of their illness and treatment. The following is a segment of the dialogue at the beginning of this group.

NURSE: Hello, everyone. I guess everybody is here that is going to be here.

MR. R.: (patient) What's your name again (to the nurse)?

NURSE: Yes, not all of you may know me; I am Miss L.; I work as a nurse in the hospital.

MRS. S.: (patient) I've seen you at the nursing station; you work during the day don't you?

NURSE: Yes, I do. (pause) Well, the real reason I've brought you together like this is so you can talk . . .

MRS. R.: (interrupts nurse) Well, I think that's a good idea. Now Harry, he doesn't talk much about himself—it worries me; everytime I want to have a serious conversation he changes the subject. I know he must be worried, but before I know it we're off talking about something that really doesn't matter. We never get anything settled . . . but I know it's hard for him, and well (gets tears in her eyes) . . .

MRS. T.: (patient) You can't be too hard on him. . . . You know having cancer—it's a terrible thing. Everything you plan for the future, all wasted, wasted! (to Mr. R.) Harry, did your doctor tell you how long you are going to have treatments?

MR. R.: (to Mrs. T. and Mr. H.) Since when does your doctor tell you anything! Listen, I'm waiting for that great cure; I'll outlive the doctor! (smiles at the group)

OTHERS: (shift uncomfortably in their seats) Silence.

MR. R.: (to Mr. H.) Who's your doctor Bill?

MR. H.: Dr. B.

MR. R.: (to Mrs. T.) Who's your doctor Mary?

MRS. T.: The same as Bill's, Dr. B.

From here the group goes on to talk about their doctors—comparing them and talking about their doctors' plans as far as they understand them. No one goes back to talking about cancer overtly, how it is a terrible thing, the great cure, or the problems of talking with your spouse about your illness. This discussion continues through most of the meeting. Just before the group terminates, the nurse reminds them that their time is up and remarks that she thinks the group "got off to a good start" and that they will meet again in 2 days. As patients and family members get ready to go back to their rooms, one patient who had been silent throughout the meeting turns and has the following conversation with the nurse.

MR. G.: I don't think I'll come anymore to these things, these group meetings. I really don't see how they will accomplish anything. (as if posing a question but at the same time making a statement)

NURSE: (busy rewinding the tape on the tape recorder) Oh, okay, uh, Mr. G., I'll tell the group you won't be coming. (without looking up)

MR. G.: Yeh, okay . . . well, I guess that's the best thing. (Mr. G. appears somewhat puzzled and leaves the nurse who is now busy rearranging the chairs in the room)

PART FOUR

Considerations for the advanced practitioner

The beginning group leader is absorbed in rudimentary nursing process issues. Nurses at this level are focused on assessment of member problems, basic group process principles, and leadership skills that will adequately equip them, for the most part, for junior coleading roles. The advanced leader who has gone beyond learning the basics of coleading and nursing process as it applies to members of a group is ready to develop more specialized skill and knowledge in issues of group work. No longer satisfied with the junior coleader role, he is motivated to establish a more autonomous function in the group—either as an equal to his social worker, psychologist, physician, or nurse coleader or as an independent leader in a group of his own design. Likewise he may be wanting to test out new research skills and special techniques. This advanced practitioner will want to know more about the subtleties of leadership, member behavior, and the effectiveness of group process as well as different techniques that can be applied to speed up group effects.

Part Four looks into these special considerations of the advanced practitioner in an attempt to identify issues and encourage experimentation and evaluation, assuming that the role of "senior" group leader requires more complex analysis and intervention.

CHAPTER 11

Coleadership and cotherapy

Introduction

Coleading in therapeutic or growth groups and cotherapy in psychotherapy groups involve two or more designated leaders or therapists in a group. Although it is usually assumed that one leader has a greater responsibility for the growth or therapeutic process of the group, the extent to which leaders share responsibility is highly variable.

Nurses have long filled the position of junior cotherapist or coleader; in fact it has not been so long since nurses have been fully recognized as capable of independent leadership or of equal coleader roles. Perhaps it was natural for nurses to fill this secondary capacity in that their knowledge and skill were limited and their general status was felt to be secondary to that of the psychologist or psychiatrist. Now, however, with the development of group leaders in graduate nursing programs, we find not only that the role of the nurse in groups has achieved an added significance and dignity but also that the role of the nurse coleader or cotherapist has taken on a new level of respectability. Nurses not only act as independent leaders in groups but also choose their own coleaders. Likewise the role of the coleader has evolved from its former junior status to a state where the coleader shares the function of leadership on an equal basis, and neither leader takes an inferior position in reference to his responsibilities in the group. This newer concept of a complementary relationship between leaders seems to hold advantages for the clients and the leaders themselves. The clients are able to profit from the combined insights and technical abilities of the leaders, and the leaders benefit from peer involvement in that they are stimulated to learn from one another.

Traditionally the cotherapy or coleadership role was adopted for the purpose of training or teaching individuals who were becoming group leaders or group therapists. As the benefits of such an approach became more obvious, leaders began to realize that coleadership or cotherapy could serve a variety of purposes. Coleading seems to enhance the experience of members because it (1) enables the group leaders to cover more area with more clients, (2) facilitates clients' working through former family conflicts via stimulation of the family group, (3) addresses special behavior or adjustment problems, for example, homosexuality and sociopathic behavior, and (4) provides actual demonstrations to clients of model patterns of relating and communicating. At the same time, cooperative effort seems to lend support and promote growth in the leaders themselves by (1) permitting the co-workers to vali-

199

date their individual perceptions and gain support for their interventions and (2) providing continual peer interaction for professional growth.

Providing broader coverage with more clients has been interpreted in a number of ways. Some leaders have taken this literally to mean that since there are two leaders in the group, there can be twice as many clients or group members. In part this argument often comes up when doubts about the economic feasibility of coleadership arise. Despite the economic implications, Godenne,[4] MacLennon,[7] and others suggest that coleaders cannot operate larger groups without becoming less effective. More precisely, the advantages of coverage that seem to occur with coleadership involve the fact that two therapists or leaders can offer more to their group than can one. Members have more than one authority figure with whom to identify and from whom to gain support, whereas with one leader fewer persons may be supported or learn through identifying with their leader.

Since there are two authority figures, similar to the primordial family situation, members are encouraged to work through typical family conflicts that may have been problematic in the past. The dual authority roles, often taken by a male and female therapist, simulate the family situation, and members react to each other as siblings and to the leaders as parental figures. This simulated situation of parents and siblings, for the leader who is particularly interested in analytically based group psychotherapy, duplicates more closely the reality of clients' long-term conflicts. According to Mintz[8] this feature encourages intense transference more quickly and therefore promotes the function of many psychoanalytically focused groups. An example of how the coleading relationship can simulate family situations and therefore be productive in helping members is illustrated in this adolescent group.

The leaders, a male child psychiatrist and female psychiatric nurse, held weekly group sessions with early adolescent boys. Each child had difficulties with dominant overbearing parents and were recognized by school authorities to have developmental or learning problems. The leaders role-modeled cooperative, collaborative behaviors in the group. Members projected expectations on them to behave as their parents but learned to their surprise that these authority figures did not demonstrate the suppressing interactions their parents did. Consequently they learned to express greater personal initiative, testing out different ways of complying to parental expectations at home.

Coleading has played a similar significant role with adjustment problems, for example, homosexuality and sociopathic adaptations. Birk, Miller, and Cohler[1] noted that coleading, when it involves a male and female therapist, is extremely useful. They found that it was important for male homosexuals to experience a group in which the male and female cotherapists worked together without dominance or exploitation of one another. They felt that the homosexual has much to relearn because he generally comes from a family in which the relationship with his mother or his father and between his parents is somewhat bizarre. In this regard a "healthy" male-female cotherapy relationship is most valuable to the experience of members.

Lastly, coleadership can serve a useful function in providing members with actual demonstrations of model patterns of relating. The interaction between co-workers can illustrate an alternative way of communicating that is useful to members. Getty and Shannon[3] imply that if the cotherapists engage in dialogue that illustrates functional communication, members may more easily change their modes of communicating by modeling them after those of the leaders. Thus the coleadership approach can be purposely employed to show members how to establish and maintain "good" interpersonal relationships.

In this case cooperation, collaboration, mutual respect, consideration, and communication skills are learned by the demonstrations of coleaders in the group. My personal experience indicates that extensive dialogue between coleaders in the context of group discussion can be extremely useful and can reduce group anxiety because it gives control back to the coleader.

An adult inpatient group session revealed tension and anxiety among group members and leaders. Coleader 1 reacted anxiously to bizarre behavior by asking the member what her head-holding behavior was about. Frustrated by other attempts to get members to talk, he began to intellectualize about the reasons for the patient's behavior as if he were going to take this episode and succeed with it. Sensing the inappropriateness of her coleader's verbal dominance in the group, coleader 2 interrupted her partner:

L_1: "Wait a minute, John. I think you are talking too much in the group right now. I think that's what Sharon (another patient) was trying to tell you too. I know I am reacting to it—can you tell me what is going on?"

L_2: "Well, I'm glad to get the feedback—what I was doing is trying to get Elaine to describe what is happening to her. It wasn't working. I'm feeling frustrated."

The group and the leaders experienced a release of tension at this time, and the pressure to resolve feelings between members also subsided. Following this exchange, members were able to give feedback to one another directly but with less pressure.

SHARON TO DAVID: "Oh, but you know I don't have to like you all the time, you know." (The group laughed as if to reinforce that negative feelings toward one another are acceptable and can be shared with respect and appreciation for the other person.)

Despite the fact that their leadership aims were not being met, this exchange between coleaders was direct and role-modeled mutual respect. The opportunity to stop the group and take stock of what was happening was facilitated by one coleader's insight and initiative to break a pattern that was being established: fruitless pursuit to change patients' behavior. Reflection enabled the group and coleaders to redirect a lost cause and freed them of the mounting tension. Members were able to demonstrate, in turn, aspects of the interaction they saw occur between the coleaders.

The purposes of coleading for the leaders themselves have received perhaps as much attention as those for clients. Most likely the reason why coleadership continues to be used even though it is obviously more expensive is that the co-workers get a great deal from working together as opposed to functioning as independent leaders. McGee and Schuman[6] express this in still another way by suggesting that all group leaders need opportunities for continual development and learning. They explain that the coleading peer involvement is an important learning experience because leaders gain an increased awareness of themselves and of their ability to work with others and a broader understanding of the skills and knowledges that can be used in group work. This experience fosters professional and personal growth and should not be foreign to any group leader despite his or her level of training and expertise.

This chance for peer contact is of further importance to the leader in the group meetings. Inside the group the leader can receive assistance and support for interventions from his co-worker. Often the coleader in the group setting provides the necessary continuity and reinforcement with interventions that make for success, that is, for situations in which themes are resolved and the process of working through members' concerns is made smooth. Having an opportunity to exchange insights and plan goals with a peer enables leaders to grow in their professional awareness and increase the overall effectiveness of interventions in the group.

Types of coleading and cotherapy relationships

The types of coleading and cotherapy relationships utilized today are probably almost as numerous as types of leadership per se. Still, three essential patterns are widely recognized and documented with some consistency in the literature. Two of these patterns suggest rather fixed and definitive functions for the leaders. The third pattern is a more flexible and individualized prescription of leader roles.

The most common and perhaps the most well-known approaches to coleading are leader-recorder (or observer) and primary-secondary leaders. These patterns require little to minimal cooperative effort on the part of the leaders and are therefore not "true" coleadership relationships despite the fact that many who use these patterns believe they are practicing coleadership or cotherapy. With the leader-recorder dyad it is clear that the sole functions of planning for and directing the group experience lies with the leader and not with the recorder (or the observer). The recorder's role is simply to listen to or to write down what is happening but not to participate. As MacLennon[7] points out, the role of the observer or recorder is misleading and usually does not work out as expected. In fact the observer or recorder is very much of a participant who may not participate verbally but who does participate nonverbally in the process of the group. According to MacLennon the observer or recorder is also an object of transference in the group. Therefore, although he may begin in a passive nondirective role capacity, he may soon be pulled into the group on a more active basis and lose his circumscribed task of simply recording and observing. It is incorrect, then, to assume that as an observer or recorder this co-worker has or can have no responsibility for what happens in the group.

The coleading or cotherapy pattern of primary-secondary leadership is almost as equally fixed and defined as the leader-observer form of coparticipation in group leadership. Primary-secondary leadership is attempted in situations where one (the secondary leader) is a trainee in group work; that is, it is a senior-junior relationship. Since this pattern is founded at the outset on the assumption that one leader has more skill and knowledge than the other—and this is usually the case—these roles are usually fixed and not always reversible even if the junior member demonstrates growth. Clearly the senior leader takes the sole responsibility for the outcome of the group and plays the major part in identifying members' needs and deciding interventions and goals. This approach to coleading is highly sheltered and protective of the trainee or junior leader. It is agreed that he needs to be free to learn from his superior so that he will be able to take a highly responsible position when he becomes the senior or primary therapist himself. It is important to note here that although the apprenticeship in group work is still employed to train group practitioners, newer methods of training include allowing trainees to learn by functioning as independent leaders at the outset or as a coleader with another trainee, as is the case in masters' programs in nursing.

A third type of leadership relationship and one that is extremely satisfying to practitioners who do not consider themselves beginners and who are willing to share leadership in groups is the egalitarian approach to coleading or cotherapy.[2] In this case the two leaders accept one another as equal in status and share the responsibility for the therapeutic process. They arrive at goals and decisions about interventions jointly and have equal opportunities to participate with individual members in the group. Differentness and disagreements between them are allowed for, and they are more free to evolve their roles in ways that are unique to them as individuals. If they wish to alternate behaviors, for example, being active or passive, directive or nondirective, they need not be concerned that they are violating their particular role function in the group, such as their function to observe only.

This relationship is satisfying not only to the coleaders themselves but also to the group, as its complimentary nature serves as an important learning experience. Since this relationship is based on mutual respect, acceptance, and shared responsibility, leaders are demonstrating to the group a healthy model of interpersonal relationships. The group has the opportunity to observe and to learn, first hand, what it takes to communicate effectively and form mutually satisfying relationships. This learning experience is extremely useful to groups of married couples and family groups where communication is dysfunctional and interactions are exploitative.

Employing cotherapy and coleadership

Different approaches to cotherapy and coleadership have been used effectively because of a variety of circumstances: the purpose of the group, the nature of the clients' problems, or the needs of the leaders to fit the particular style of coparticipation. Coleadership as junior-senior roles will always be an important means for training novices in group work. This is because the junior member does need to take a less active role if he is to concentrate on learning the many things he needs to know to lead a group. Other forms of cotherapy may be important, however, in groups of homosexuals, groups of delinquents, groups of married couples, and groups that are analytic in focus.

In a group of homosexuals a male-female cotherapy situation with either the junior-senior pattern or egalitarian pattern is past. The male-female relationship in which the female takes on the less dominant junior position decreases threats to members of an exploitative mother, according to Birk, Miller, and Cohler.[1] In addition, however, if both therapists work as an egalitarian team, members relearn what a relationship between male and female can be.

Members reexperience new models

Since delinquents and sociopathic persons need to rework or work through "bad" and "good" features of parental figures, the type of cotherapy relationship may not be so important as the responses these leaders are able to evoke by their individual personalities. The coleaders may be male-female, male-male, or female-female. More important is the fact that one leader represents the "bad" mother or father and the other, the "good" parental figure. Under these conditions members can work through their feelings and resolve their conflicts about their parents more quickly. An example of this possibility was given earlier in a description of an early adolescent group.

Leader regains control and direction

In some cases, as in a group of young children or a group of delinquent teenagers, a form of coleadership is important for a practical reason. In children's groups it often happens that a coleader is needed to contain and control the group. This is especially true if these children are likely to act out their feelings and frustrations, and therefore produce a great deal of strain on one therapist, or be physically assaultive.

One female leader in a children's group expressed confusion and exasperation when she seemed to be getting nowhere in the group. She was attempting to use a behavioral modification approach and direct members to describe what they wanted from a friend. Although the topic was well defined, because of the chaos in the group —children hitting one another, interrupting the person talking, shifting in their chairs, and teasing one another—her purpose was not being achieved. She had so many behaviors to hold in check that she found herself rewarding undesired behavior, letting "good" children leave the group and having disruptive children stay and talk. The stress on this one leader was overwhelming, and no way out seemed to be forthcoming until of course the natural ending of the group because time was up.

If she had had a coleader there would have been several options open to her. One of course would be that she could focus on the task, and her coleader could manage behavior reinforcement. Another option would have been that her coleader could interrupt her frantic attempts to direct the group and guide the group to take on some of the burden of making each other adhere to the group task.

Members learn new ways from models

In groups of married couples and groups with multiple families, as noted previously, an egalitarian approach by male-female cotherapists is most appropriate. Clients of both sexes have like-sexed therapists with whom they can identify. In addition couples can see the co-workers relate to each other on an adult-adult level. Their own problems may parallel issues of the cotherapy relationship that have been worked out successfully by the therapists, for example, shared responsibility, mutual respect, and interdependency. The therapists illustrate how authority can be distributed effectively and how both members of the therapeutic team can allow the other to grow within the relationship—a situation that strongly parallels the needs of many couples and families.

The following description of cotherapy dialogue illustrates the leaders' modeling respect for each others' purpose and demonstrates potential impact on members' interacting supportively in the group:

L_1: "Let's take a problem you are having right now—and discuss that." (directing focus)

Group does not stay on the subject.

L_2: "Going back to what Bob (L_1) said—what specifically bothers you about your medication?" (compliments L_1's intervention and shows respect for L_1's purpose)

Group takes up a specific topic again. Near the end of the group:

L_1: "Gwen (L_2) did you want to pass out the form now?" (opens space for L_2's needs; acknowledges with respect)

Members gain insight into conflicts

Groups led for the specific purpose of developing members' insights into deep-seated conflicts, for example, analytically focused therapy groups, would seem to benefit from a junior-senior cotherapy approach. The purpose of this group is to bring to members' awareness the basic archaic family relationships that affect members' current level of functioning and adjustment. The male-female, senior-junior form of cotherapy parallels the typical parental model of authority. It intentionally facilitates and speeds up the transference of reactions to the therapists, which can then be observed by the leaders and worked through by individuals in the group. The feelings, attitudes, and expectations projected onto the therapists as authority figures are discussed as possible remnants of former relationships with parents of both sexes. When transference is important for the success of the group, it is important that there be a coleader who can suggest alternative interpretations to the reactions of members in the group.

Despite the effectiveness of coleadership or cotherapy and the many purposes it can serve, it is not without problems. These problems seem to arise even more frequently when therapists attempt to utilize an egalitarian approach, since tasks of continuity and coordination become more complicated.

One of the most common problems any pair of co-workers encounters is working at cross-purposes in the group. Since leaders may differ in their ideas about the objectives of the group or the nature of their client population, in their philosophy, or in their specific training in group work, the potential threat exists that their interventions will not always fit and therefore will conflict. In essence their complementary relationship is not complementary in action.

In addition to the problem of coordination created by the differences in leaders' outlooks is the problem of operating in the group when one does not understand or know how to work with the other. There may be confusion about who is going to do what and when. If the leaders are confused, they will more than likely confuse the group and increase members' anxiety. Group members need to believe that the therapists know what they are doing and that they can direct them successfully in reaching their goals. Most leaders can sense this dependence of members on them and become uncomfortable with their own disorganization.

A third and extremely important problem between co-workers is their failure to give enough attention to the progress of their own relationship. As Heilfron[5] suggests, co-workers frequently assume that their focus should be on their clients to the point that they ignore their own relationship. They assume that their interaction in the group will be characterized by unconditional acceptance, loyalty, and objectivity. Frequently, feelings such as jealousy, resentment, or dependence may occur and not be worked out sufficiently because the coleaders are too busy working on the group's problems. Particularly in a junior-senior cotherapy relationship co-workers may develop transference reactions to one another and not realize what is happening until (1) one leader takes over and the second leader allows him to dominate, (2) one leader supports the client against the other leader, or (3) one leader tries to prove he is stronger, more skillful, or "nicer" than the other and manipulates the group into coming to this conclusion. In these instances the leader who is transferring feelings and expectations to his partner may be looking at his co-worker as a father or mother figure along with the group (that is, acting as a sibling) or may be looking at his co-worker as a spouse (as in the client fantasy). Most of the time transference situations such as these are out of the leaders' immediate awareness.

To minimize the problems that coleadership or cotherapy can present and at the same time reap the benefits of such a satisfying approach to group work, several provisions can be made.

Perhaps one of the most important facts for coleaders and cotherapists to keep in mind when they are leading a group is that the relationship between them influences the group and therefore plays an integral part in the outcome of the group experience for members. When co-workers avoid looking at the relationship between one another in favor of a focus on "the group's problems," they minimize an important aspect of the group. It is natural for them to wonder about how the other sees them and to be puzzled about what the other is doing, as well as to develop a variety of strong emotions about their peer. Coleaders must view the total interaction of the group in its complexity: as Heilfron[5] suggests, what happens in the group is a result of the communication between leaders, of the interactions between leaders and members, and of communication among members. If co-workers recognize the complexity of this interactional network, they are more likely to give a concerted effort to analyzing and building on the relationship between them.

McGee and Schuman[6] along this same line indicate that co-workers usually have several opportunities to function together and should take advantage of these situations to build on their relationship. They can meet to screen potential group members and will attend group sessions together; in addition they may meet to rehash the group sessions and may be supervised jointly by an outside person. In addition to these contacts, where they are concerned with looking at the group, they may also attend agency meetings or social events where the other is present. At any of these times they may recognize that they are facing certain issues in their relationship which may cause some tension. Rather than negate the significance of these clues, they should take a serious look at what is going on between them. They should realize that any relationship, even their cotherapy relationship, goes through certain phases or stages, for example, of inclusion, control, and affection. They cannot expect to be completely complementary or cohesive at first.

Since co-workers need time to assess and develop themselves as a functional unit and because they are virtually strangers at the outset, designated times should be set aside for them to meet alone and together with an outside person. Their participation in hash and rehash sessions is extremely important. They can plan and evaluate methods of working together and their mutual roles. This helps to resolve some of the beginning mechanical problems of working together. In these sessions co-workers can build on a common foundation or understanding about the group and the needs of the clients, as well as become aware of areas of differences, for example, in their perceptions of goals for the group and their style of leadership. In coleading, as opposed to independent leadership, timing of interventions and follow-through can be more of a problem. If coleaders formulate a plan of action ahead of time in which they decide on the way to handle certain concerns of members and the priorities for intervention, working together in the group will be facilitated.

In addition to the hash and rehash sessions that coleaders hold between themselves, it is advisable for them to meet periodically, if not regularly, with a supervisor. This third person can be utilized to help the coleaders assess the nature of their relationship and to help them envision how their own interaction affects the group and individuals within the group. The supervisor can detect any transference or countertransference the leaders are having between themselves or with clients. Emotion-ladened issues of control, dominance, affection, or intimacy between coleaders can take on greater clarity when there is an objective outsider to identify and isolate the issues. Likewise coleaders can learn how their battle over which leader is going to direct the group, for example, can cause members to play one leader against the other or can stimulate favoritism in the group. When they are caught up in these complex relationship problems, it helps to have a supervisor who will lend support and at the same time help them become aware of and deal with the issues.

In sessions with my own supervisees I frequently spend more time focusing on their relationship than what was talked about in their last group session. The reasons are multiple. One, the problems the supervisees are having often give clues about the covert process of the group. When a coleading dyad is trying to develop an egalitarian relationship, I often spend time reinforcing mutual respect, encouraging them to validate communication with one another and express their feelings directly to each other. The relationship I help create in the supervisory session facilitates leader modeling in the group itself.

If a supervisor is not available, tape-recorded group sessions may be used to aid the coleaders in looking more objectively at what is going on in the group and at the

Names of group leaders _____
_____
_____

GROUP LEADER QUESTIONNAIRE

Session no. _____
Date _____

Please complete a Group Leader Questionnaire following each session of your group.

1. How many members did you expect to appear at this session? _____
2. How many actually appeared? _____
3. Group cohesiveness may be defined as the extent to which the group experiences a sense of solidarity or "we-ness." How cohesive would you judge your group to be at this session? (Please check response that describes your group.)

Highly cohesive___   Moderately cohesive___   Slightly cohesive___   Not at all cohesive___   Unable to determine___

Comments:
_____
_____
_____

4. Did members demonstrate high levels of self-disclosure of personal feelings, thoughts, fears, and concerns?

Yes, very high___   Yes, moderately high___   No, only slightly___   Not at all self-disclosing___   Unable to determine___

Comments:
_____
_____

5. Briefly state what you think were the main overt (content) themes of your group (that is, what did they talk about?).
_____
_____

6. Briefly state what you think were the main covert themes of your group (that is, what do you think was going on in the interactions between members or between members and leader[s]?).
_____
_____
_____

7. Which adjectives describe the chief way(s) members responded to you? (Please circle those that describe your members.)

Compliant	Noncompliant
Friendly	Hostile
Cooperative	Resistant
Trusting	Suspicious

If others, please specify:

_____   _____   _____

_____   _____   _____

_____   _____   _____

8. What would you judge was the affect or mood(s) of your group this session? _____

_____

9. What is your feeling(s) in response to what happened in your group? (This question can be answered by the leaders separately if they feel differently about the session. Please feel free to say what you truly feel.)

Leader (Name _____):

_____

_____

_____

Leader (Name _____):

_____

_____

_____

feelings they have toward one another. In addition the tape will indicate to them how they may be distorting what is happening due to feelings they have about the group, their roles, or their relationship.

When tape recordings and the time it takes to rehash these recordings are not feasible, the leaders may design a questionnaire to facilitate their discussions of salient points about each group session. The boxed material on pp. 208-209 is an example of such a questionnaire that my coleader and I developed for use in an affective-disorder group to keep as an ongoing analysis of process and content in our sessions. The reader, to zero in more directly on coleading issues, might add questions such as: What problems arose in the coleadership relationship? In what cases, if any, were coleadership interventions operating at cross-purposes? In what areas, if any, do the coleaders disagree or agree about philosophy, purpose, or assessment?

Choosing a coleader

In the literature on coleading and cotherapy, some attention is given to the proper pairing of co-workers. Is it important, for example, that coleaders know each other ahead of time? Must coleaders respect, trust, and like one another? Are there certain characteristics leaders should have in common? Or how, and to what degree, should they differ? Although it is generally agreed that coleaders should probably have a beginning potential for mutual respect and trust, it is felt that they need not know each other ahead of time. In some cases a previous relationship between co-workers is not a good reason to pair leaders. Coleaders who have been friends or acquaintances usually have much to work out prior to their cooperative involvement in the group. Two coleaders, for example, who have worked together in an agency deal with cooperation, competition, and intimacy in other contexts. Their history of resolving these issues may or may not delay a healthy coleadership alliance.

Most group practitioners believe that all differences between coleaders should not be eliminated. On the contrary, clients need to see that persons in authority can be different and still work together. Also more clients may be able to relate to or identify with the leaders if these practitioners do differ in personality or philosophy. Too often members assume that differentness and disagreement is "bad," especially between those in authority. When co-workers are chosen so that they differ from one another along certain lines, the group has an important lesson to learn, namely, how to get along with people different from themselves. They learn by example from the coleaders how both can be allowed to grow in their unique ways. Coleaders' ability to provide a model for resolution of differences and disagreements is an important element in teaching clients in the group.

While differences between coleaders are helpful, it is important to continually identify how they impact on the group. As a common practice I encourage my supervisees to complete a FIRO-B[9] measure. The FIRO-B clarifies basic personality differences that affect their responses in group. Whereas it is not the only scale that can be useful in highlighting areas of conflict between coleaders, it is a useful, brief analysis that has direct implications for group interaction.

At the outset when leaders are pairing to form coleader dyads and at a selected time in the introductory stage of the group, coleaders should complete this personal analysis. The scale will indicate each leader's needs for expressing and getting from others inclusion, control, and affection. In cases where coleaders are clearly not complementary, this fact is surely to show up in group interaction and leaders' ability to work together.

For example, one of my coleader dyads was experiencing difficulty in coordinating mutual efforts inside the group. One leader remained relatively passive in the group, letting the other lead and initiate most interventions. Tension was building between them, but it was not until we discussed the results of the FIRO-B that we saw and understood what the problem was.

The passive leader's score on control indicated that she was below the mean in expressing control but well above average in wanting control from others. The active leader's score on control indicated that she did not wish to control others and was lower than average on wanting others to control her. In discussing the fact that the active leader was exerting direction on the group but probably did not want to do this as much as she had, we discovered that she was trying to fill in the gap because her coleader was not directive at all. She was unhappy with the burden of doing more than her share. Up to this time the passive leader had not realized the bind her coleader was in. Recognizing that the passive-active positions they had solidified in the group gave neither of them room to grow—and probably affected the group adversely—they decided to equalize the passive-active aspects of their roles. The passive leader experimented with more directive techniques, and the active leader paused before intervening so that her coleader would have a chance to intervene more frequently.

Perhaps the most important common denominator in deciding the selection of coleaders to work together is their ability and willingness to work as a team. It is extremely important that cotherapists be flexible and have a beginning understanding of how to relate to others in a complementary manner. If they are flexible about priorities in their interaction and about their own roles in the group, they are more likely to adjust to the need of deciding on things jointly. At the same time they are less likely to be anxious or purposely disruptive with regard to their peer's position in the group. Although this is an essential ingredient of the egalitarian approach to coleading, it is also necessary for junior-senior and leader-observer forms of coleading.

Coleading, like independent leadership, is not appropriate for every leader or therapist. Every practitioner should not expect to operate as a coleader, nor feel inadequate if he does his best when he is leading independently. As we have noted several times in this chapter, coleading or cotherapy is not easier; it is extremely complex and requires much effort to make it work effectively.

REFERENCES

1. Birk, L., Miller, E., and Cohler, B.: Group psychotherapy for homosexual men by male-female co-therapists. In Sager, E., and Kaplin, H., editors: Progress in group and family therapy, New York, 1972, Brunner/Mazel, pp. 680-711.
2. Getty, C., and Shannon, A.: Co-therapy as an egalitarian relationship, University of California Medical Center, Graduate Department, Psychiatric Nursing, Reprint, San Francisco, 1967.
3. Getty, C., and Shannon, A.: Nurses as co-therapists in a family-therapy setting, Perspect. Psychiatr. Care **5:**36-47, 1967.
4. Godenne, G. D.: Outpatient adolescent group psychotherapy. I. A review of the literature on the use of co-therapists, psychodrama, and parent group therapy, Am. J. Psychother. **18:** 584-593, 1964.
5. Heilfron, M.: Co-therapy: the relationship between therapists, Int. J. Group Psychother. **19:**366-381, 1969.
6. McGee, I., and Schuman, B.: The nature of the co-therapy relationship, Int. J. Group Psychother. **20:**25-36, 1970.
7. MacLennon, B.: Co-therapy, Int. J. Group Psychother. **15:**154-166, 1965.
8. Mintz, E. E.: Transference in co-therapy groups, J. Consult. Psychol. **27:**34-39, 1963.

9. Schutz, W.: FIRO: a 3-dimensional theory of interpersonal behavior, New York, 1958, Holt, Rinehart & Winston.

SUGGESTED READINGS

Davis, F. B., and Lohr, N. E.: Special problems with the use of co-therapists in group psychotherapy, Int. J. Group Psychother. **21:**143-157, 1971.

Farhood, L.: Choosing a partner for co-therapy, Perspect. Psychiatr. Care **8:**177-179, 1975.

Gans, R.: Group co-therapists and the therapeutic situation: a critical evaluation, Int. J. Group Psychother. **12:**82-87, 1962.

Heckel, R.: The nurse as co-therapist in group psychotherapy, Perspect. Psychiatr. Care **2:** 18-22, 1964.

Kassoff, A.: Advantages of multiple therapists in a group of severely acting-out adolescent boys, Int. J. Group Psychother. **8:**70-75, 1958.

Krasner, J., Feldman, B., Liff, Z., et al.: Observing the observers, Int. J. Group Psychother. **14:** 214-217, 1964.

Linden, M.: The significance of dual leadership in gerontologic group psychotherapy, Int. J. Group Psychother. **4:**262-273, 1954.

Mintz, E. E.: Special values of co-therapists in group psychotherapy, Int. J. Group Psychother. **13:**127-132, 1963.

Pine, I., Todd, W., and Boenheim, C.: Special problems of resistance in co-therapy groups, Int. J. Group Psychother. **13:**354-362, 1963.

Rabin, H.: How does co-therapy compare with regular group therapy? Am. J. Psychother. **21:** 244-255, 1967.

Rosenbaum, M.: Co-therapy in comprehensive group psychotherapy, Baltimore, 1971, The Williams & Wilkins Co.

Weinstein, I.: Guidelines on the choice of a co-therapist, Psychother. Theory Res. Prac. **8:** 301-303, 1971.

Whitaker, L., and Napier, A.: A conversation about co-therapy. In Ferber, A., et al: Book of family therapy, Boston, 1973, Houghton Mifflin Co.

CHAPTER 12

Typing behavior

Introduction

The simplified concepts of group relations and group behavior as "leader-follower" have undergone much revision. Through the study and research of psychosocial theorists and functional analysts the number of possible member roles or behaviors has grown from these two basic concepts (leader and follower) to twenty-seven or more roles members can assume in a group setting. Some of these roles or behaviors are conceptualized along the lines of what the group needs from its participants; still others include concepts of deviant role behavior, as well as general character analysis. For example, these roles encompass such things as group task activities, group development activities, and "antigroup" activities. In the case of antigroup behavior, members clearly deviate from those behaviors the leader feels should be the norm in the group.

The growing sophistication about group behavior has made the traditional leader-follower concepts outdated and irrelevant. In addition, knowledge about the variety of behaviors that occur in groups and how they combine in group interaction produces a more liberal attitude in our expectations of participants. If antigroup behavior is in fact regarded as commonplace, leaders are somewhat less annoyed when it occurs. Also, if one anticipates encountering a variety of behaviors from participants, he is less likely to consider any one behavior as especially deviant, unacceptable, or foreign. Still, equally important is the idea that when we can look at clear and subtle changes in individuals' behaviors, we can predict and test out theories of behavior alteration. Our predictions may be based on the effects of group process, the interaction of certain members with others, and the impact of the leaders on selected behavior patterns.

Despite the growing sophistication about group behavior, there remain some areas of ambiguity on which theorists continue to vacillate. These issues revolve around the question of how behaviors should be interpreted: (1) Is an individual's behavior in a group transient or is it highly constant and predictable in any given group situation? (2) Can members' behaviors be sufficiently described in terms of group needs or do they reflect individual needs and desires to a larger extent? (3) As the group grows, will members' behavior change? And, likewise, does the growth of the group depend on certain changes in behavior of its members? Although theorists are prepared to accept the fact that certain roles or behaviors appear and reappear with unmistakable regularity, they are not in total agreement on how to look at these

213

behaviors and why they occur in the first place. As a result of the classic findings of the Hawthorne experiment in 1927 on the conditions of environment that affect behavior and of the Lewin, Lippitt, and White findings in 1937 to 1940 on the relationship between group atmosphere, styles of leadership, and behavior of group members, it is no longer certain that members' behaviors are solely the result of their unique personalities. Still the extent to which the group as a whole (or interpersonal interplay) influences participants' activities has not been clarified.

These issues and questions arise whenever the group leader or therapist is faced with assessing his group and deciding what should be done to enhance overall development and the individual growth of each participant. If one believes, for example, that members' behaviors are highly constant and fixed and that a dominator in one group will continue to dominate in other groups, his approach may differ from that which he might employ if he understood that his style of leadership or some other factor in the group is causing this individual to behave as he is.

There are sound reasons, then, why theorists continue to analyze, identify, and isolate types of group behavior. The ability to predict, plan for, and control group behavior depends on knowledge of why certain behaviors occur and the perceptions of what they entail. This ability has been sought by those in fields other than nursing, such as law enforcement, social work, and education. For the nurse group psychotherapist or nurse group leader a knowledge of group behavior and the interaction of roles is extremely important in assessing the need for specific interventions. The nurse group leader, based on assessments of behaviors in the group and objectives for participants, decides the course of interaction.

Although areas of ambiguity exist and are frustrating to the practitioner, they do in fact indicate the wealth of researchable questions enveloped in group work.

The following discussion describes various conceptual models that can be employed in identifying behavior of group participants. These models primarily originate from either a group dynamics or psychotherapeutic-psychiatric theoretical framework. After the various behaviors in these models are described, the implications of such models for the role of the nurse will be considered. What behaviors are important and why will be examined more specifically, in terms of the nurse's role in fostering group development and individual growth.

Assuming a role or stereotyped position in a group setting is a means for the individual to establish an identity. It is a means of answering the question: Who am I and what will I be in this group? In part it is a reaction to the group, but also it is a reflection of himself as he understands others see him. After he has established a position based on reactions to the group and perceptions of others' expectations, the individual's behavior patterns may become solidified. Essentially he may continue to act according to how others see him. At this point, behavior is more easily identified and categorized. And, despite the fact that behavior can be seen as depicting various positions in many dimensions, for example, active or passive, independent or dependent, hindering or helpful, antagonistic or protagonistic, leading or following, an individual will come to be known rather narrowly as one type or another, such as passive-dependent or hindering-antagonistic.

Few group enthusiasts have resisted the temptation to classify and type human behavior. Group dynamics and psychotherapeutic theorists are the most active in typing behaviors in groups. This discussion will deal with several frameworks that lend themselves to typing behavior.

Group dynamics viewpoints

Underlying various group dynamics viewpoints of group behavior is a concept of group development. These theorists maintain that each group goal appears to have a parallel set of required group functions. Members' activities that contribute to or deny the performance of these functions can be typed and referred to as behaviors (1) contributing to the maintenance of the group, (2) moving the group toward its goals, or (3) helping the individual achieve his own personal goals (ego-oriented) irrespective of the needs of the group as a whole.[4] In this sense then the alleged goals of the group may be seen to exert influence over members and thus steer and activate behavior along more or less constructive lines.

The most widely used and classic concept of behavior as functional roles in the group is that of Benne and Sheats.[1] Benne and Sheats described the three types of functions mentioned above, which encompass several roles or behavioral patterns.

The behaviors associated with group locomotion toward group goals are those of seeking information, giving information, and recording. They include the initiator, the information or opinion seeker, the information or opinion giver, the coordinator, the evaluator, the energizer, and the procedural technician. These task functionaries help the group identify and solve problems associated with the goals of the group. They are the rational administrators of the group who clearly relate as leaders from time to time.

Behaviors seen as contributing to the maintenance of the group are those of encouraging participation, harmonizing between persons, and expediting communication. They include the encourager, the harmonizer, the compromiser, the standard setter, the group commentator, and the typical "follower" who agrees to go along with the majority. More passive in respect to group problem solving, these persons add the necessary component of emotionality and standardization. They keep the group going and at the same time keep members in check so that relationships in the group are maintained and enhanced.

Lastly, behaviors that work for the attainment of personal goals only are those that express aggression or that seek action on personal interests at the expense of the group as a whole. They include the aggressor, the blocker, the recognition or help seeker, the playboy, the self-confessor, the dominator, and the special interest pleader. These persons usually behave in ways irrelevant to either the group task or the problems of building and maintaining relationships in the group. Since they are seen as basically destructive or disruptive, they are discouraged as much as possible.

Underlying this conceptual model of individuals' behavior in groups is a democratic value orientation. Clearly members are succumbing to the desires of the majority if they relinquish personal need satisfaction. Along this same line, behaviors not clearly directed toward group goals or maintenance of the group are undesirable, deviant, and should be altered. The corrective mechanism here is to keep individuals from straying too far from the path of the group goal or the "good" of the total group.

There are many assumptions and ideas worthy of research and documentation within this theoretical framework. Following are some of the most important:

1. To what extent can behavior in the group be classified as either constructive or destructive to group goals?
2. To what extent do individuals remain in one or the other role function throughout the group?
3. To what extent do the efforts of group leaders to keep individuals aligned with group goals influence change in the individual's personality makeup?

Psychotherapeutic and psychiatric viewpoints

The communication theory of Satir[6] and the modified analytic theory of Berne[2] present interesting concepts applicable for typing the behavior of individuals and dyads in groups.

Satir, in addition to specifying persons as functional, dysfunctional, or model communicators, goes one step further in identifying behavioral syndromes that can occur in groups or dyads of individuals. We described one syndrome when we discussed the mind-reading phenomenon in Chapter 10. Satir gives a basic account of the implications of these syndromes for the individual, which is most helpful.

Satir's premise is that the behavioral syndromes that can occur between individuals in groups are often caused by a lack of self-esteem or self-respect. Participants may be attempting to preserve or otherwise enhance a relatively poor self-concept when relating in the group. In essence the behavior patterns we see may be defenses against the realization of low self-esteem. When this behavior prevents the establishment of effective communication, it is viewed as deviating from the leader's objectives for persons and therefore necessitates leader intervention and change on the part of participants.

Four basic syndromes that have not yet been discussed and that Satir describes are the fragility, teeter-totter, blackmail, and war syndromes. These behavior patterns are indicative of dysfunctional communication and faulty interpersonal relationships, as well as of low self-esteem.

The fragility syndrome[6] occurs between persons who cannot take the risk of looking clearly and objectively at themselves and their behavior. Basically they are afraid of giving and receiving feedback. One fears that the other is weak and unable to accept what he might do or say. In turn he views himself as fragile and likely to fall apart. Both parties are potential victims of possible disaster. In response to these beliefs, persons will (1) avoid getting feedback on issues that are important to them, (2) avoid giving feedback on issues important to others, (3) refer to themselves or others as being "vulnerable," "little," "weak," or "sick," and (4) become extremely uncomfortable when emotion-ladened topics in the group bring members in conflict with one another.

The teeter-totter syndrome[6] is a case in which persons engage in out-and-out battle. Persons participating in this syndrome communicate directly and openly but pull at each other so that no understanding occurs. One gets the feeling that only mental or verbal gymnastics with no logical or fruitful end point are being played out. These individuals (1) usually shout or talk loudly in order to present their side of an issue or problem, (2) frequently interrupt one another as they get more and more convinced that they are "right," and (3) make it virtually impossible for anyone else to interject a comment. Observing the interplay between these persons, one receives the impression that there is no single monopolizer but more than one at work at the same time in the group. Each fights for both his time to "take the floor" and his need to be "right," "correct," or most astute.

The blackmail and war syndromes[6] are additional interactional patterns that frequently appear in groups, especially between members with bonds developed prior to their coming to the group, for example, with married couples or families. The war syndrome occurs between members who have a conflict of interests. The battle they wage is often to decide who will have control in the situation—who will win or who will decide for the group. They confuse the issue with the desire to come out on top, to lose as little as possible, and to preserve as much as possible. Persons engaged in war (1) attempt to divide the group as to "what side are you on," thereby developing an offensive team, (2) disregard issues and stress alliances, loyalties, and "who is right," and (3) firmly state their position and attempt to elicit others' reactions based on this position, thereby giving the impression of a cleavage in the group. Persons who participate in blackmail, like those who lead war and relate in terms of other dysfunctional syndromes, truly suffer from low self-esteem. Blackmail[6] occurs especially, however, when persons fear accountability for their actions.

Blackmailers, as we know, abdicate responsibility for their behavior; they are made to do "bad" things by others. The fact that others did not cooperate with their demands is the reason they acted the way they did, not because they wanted to. Blackmailers usually show that they (1) are basically "good" people, but (2) are frequently "victims" of circumstances, and (3) are willing to change if something else occurs to appease or placate them. They continually put others on the defensive by threatening: "If you . . . then I will," or "You better not . . ." (the consequences are not spelled out but are implicit and severe enough to stop the other person). The blackmailer makes it clear to the group as a whole and to individuals in the group that his position is highly dependent on what happens and how he is treated, thereby putting everyone on edge.

Along the same lines as Satir, Eric Berne has also identified various roles or behaviors that have significance for group interaction. As was pointed out in Chapter 6, Berne's theory of transactional analysis rests with identifying individuals' behaviors in terms of child, parent, and adult. Essentially individuals are acting out one of these roles when they interact with one another. In addition to these roles, Berne describes other various behavior patterns that every group leader should be aware of. These are "I'm only trying to help you," which is frequently played by the helping person or leader, and peasant and wooden-leg, which are demonstrated by their clients.

"I'm only trying to help you"[2,3] is enacted by group leaders who claim that their role is strictly a helping one and therefore whatever they do is justified. Frequently the leader may demonstrate this behavior in that he readily gives advice to his group. He rarely questions his motives or the adequacy of his advice because giving such advice or interpretations is what he sees to be the modus operandi of the helping profession. The complement position of the client or the group is "Oh, how wonderful our leader," or "There is nothing you can do." The leader's position denies the group its opportunity to solve its own problems and to account for its own success and failures. Much more important to the group leader is verification of his own adequacy as a "helper" rather than proof of the strength of his clients. In most cases the leader does not succeed because members fail to take advice or fail to act on the advice correctly and therefore reinforce the attitude of the leader that members are truly incompetent.

Peasant[2] is played by the group or individuals in the group who respond to the leader as an awesome authority who knows more, does more, and succeeds more frequently than anyone else they know. The group may be overcome with admiration for the education or skill or both of the leader. The leader is so impressed with such expression that he does not realize there has been virtually no change in members, even though he has administered his best techniques. The whole point is that if the leader is led astray by these expressions, he may not have an opportunity to seriously look at the group's problems and actually do something about them. If he recognizes this interpersonal trap, he needs to consider why it is occurring. The leader must decide whether this game is played innocently—whether the group is honestly taken aback with his talents—or whether members are utilizing the "Gee, you're great" technique to keep the leader from giving *their* problems serious attention. As Berne suggests, if the game is being played innocently, then the leader may want to let it go until the group is stronger before using countermeasures. If the act is premeditated, however, the leader should probably present the group with its deception early. The group should be made aware of the position they have put the leader in and the obvious consequences; for example, the group spends so much time admiring the leader that it never gets around to looking at its own problems. Once the group recognizes this maneuver, members are more likely to abandon the peasant behavior in pursuit of looking inward and tackling problems.

Wooden-leg is another role taken by clients. In a group setting the leader may be confronted with protests; for example, "How can you expect me (us) to change when I (we) have been sick for so long?" or "I'm too far gone to ever get back to normal (the usual, my old strong self, and so on)." The once disturbed client or highly rigid personality will play this game in a group, especially when he feels pressure from the group or from the leader to change. By claiming wooden-leg, that he is too young or too fragile, the individual or the group excuses itself from outrageous, unacceptable, unexpected, or irrational behavior. Their handicap (age, background, emotional disturbance, or lack of knowledge and skill in relating to people) has put them in a position where they are unable to fulfill the objectives of the leader for the group as a whole or for their individual development. This disability, although frequently real, may be exaggerated or even purely imaginary. If the leader believes the plight of the group or that of the individual member, he will tend to overprotect them. If this happens, the group will get nowhere and the leader may become increasingly distressed with their disability. Futility reigns and the group or the leader may decide to disband early because "It's no use." However, if the leader can decipher what has occurred and pose the alternative "What do you expect of yourselves, irrespective of your limitations? (giving time for the group to answer the question), the game is likely to be disrupted, instead of the group itself. Members are encouraged to look at themselves, not in terms of what the leader expects of them but in terms of what they expect of themselves. Having arrived at some answers, they will be obliged to live up to these expectations or face the realization that living with their disability is more advantageous. Either outcome is a fruitful learning experience for the group and an important basis for future intervention on the part of the leader.

The concepts and frameworks of Berne and Satir also contain a wealth of researchable problems. The whole premise of Satir's theory that communication syndromes appear with an onset of a threat to the self-esteem should be documented. In case study 1, reported in Chapter 10, I documented the occurrence of syndromes as they related to threats to individuals inside the group. More documentation of the arousal and release of syndrome behavior is needed.

Berne's theory that syndromes or games are linked with secondary "payoffs" is still another concept needing documentation. To what extent are "payoffs" the reason for pursuing learned patterns? To what extent are these patterns rhythmic and unconsciously reinforced? To what extent does leader interruption and group pressure effect sustained changes in individual's patterns?

Implications for leader intervention

Generally, if the role of the nurse group leader or therapist is to foster the development of the group as a whole and to enhance the growth of individuals in the group, behavior patterns have special meaning. By reviewing those behaviors previously discussed, it can be seen that several of these patterns should come under the scrutiny of the nurse, suggesting the need for specific interventions.

From the viewpoint of the group dynamics model the roles of deviants or ego-oriented persons in the group need attention. Those who pursue individual interests at the expense of group problem-solving needs for development and maintenance, clearly deviate from the behavioral norms decided on by the leader who has a democratic value orientation. Those who exhibit certain behaviors, such as aggressors, blockers, recognition seekers, self-confessors, dominators, and special interest pleaders, interfere with the group's development. The nurse, as well as other members, has an implied obligation to alter these behaviors, thereby making individuals' contributions more helpful to the needs of the group. Members should generally be guided to set goals, move toward these goals, and improve the quality of total group interaction. When these objectives are fulfilled, group growth and cohesion are more likely to occur.

From a psychotherapeutic viewpoint, patterned responses or behaviors have an added significance. The nurse is concerned not only with the behavior of participants for the "good" of the group but also with behaviors as they depict the health and well-being of individuals and dyads within the group. To the group psychotherapist many of these patterned behaviors or stereotyped roles are acted out by individuals on an unconscious basis.[5] Patterned behaviors can represent certain defensive modes of coping with a group situation. When an individual utilizes his existing repertoire of behaviors, he gets others to respond in a fashion that is customary and safe for him. If others respond as expected, there is no need to change.

The nurse's role with behavioral syndromes (war and blackmail) and with game playing (peasant) is to create an environment in the group where change in these patterns is feasible. To do this the nurse must (1) decrease threats to members' self-esteem, (2) increase opportunities for security in the group, and (3) initiate feedback exchange from which members can learn about the origins and effects of their behavior, as well as experiment with new behaviors.

In this sense, then, the task of the nurse leader is to do away with all stereotyped, fixed behavior responses—whether they are for the "good" of the group or not. The assumption here is that, although certain behavior patterns may be useful to the group and to the individual—at least initially, members will grow if they are free to relinquish rigid patterns and develop themselves on several dimensions with reference to their ability to lead or follow, to be active or passive, or to hinder or help. Rigid behavior patterns are viewed as symptoms of anxiety, guilt, and low self-esteem. If persons were free from such feelings, they would no longer react in terms of distinct behavioral patterns.

Decreasing threats to members' self-esteem

Behind many behavior patterns is the objective to minimize threat to one's self-esteem. Members may interpret many comments as direct attacks on their self-esteem. In light of this phenomenon, it is known that members engage in various game-playing roles and syndromes tending to support their self-esteem or self-worth, often at the cost of the other's self-esteem.

Several things the nurse can do to minimize threats to individuals and therefore decrease the need for patterned responses are (1) handling emotion-ladened discussions with care, (2) switching to less difficult issues when the interaction and communication on one topic gets blocked, (3) setting (and reminding members about) rules for interaction that do not permit anyone to profit through the defeat of another person, (4) showing the capability of moving the group toward its stated objectives, and (5) avoiding bias on taking sides in an argument. The nurse's nonjudgmental attitude, sensitivity, and ability to intervene and redirect members along more interpersonally constructive lines provides the reassurance members need to relinquish fears of threats to their self-worth.

Increasing opportunities for security in the group

Since many behavior patterns are a result of attempts to preserve self-esteem, it is important to decrease threats in the group and at the same time to take an active role in increasing members' sense of security. There are several things the leader can do to make members feel more secure. A consistent approach will provide a certain structure to the group and put members at ease; however, the nurse can (1) focus on giving support and confidence that will make members less anxious about their group experience and what will occur, (2) illustrate how what the leader does has some underlying meaning in terms of the group objective and what members need to learn, (3) show the purpose for the group and the ability to guide the group safely and effectively toward this goal, and (4) point out that nothing disastrous is going to happen to the group as a whole despite the fears and reservations individuals may have brought with them.

The leader should realize that numerous opportunities to project ideology and philosophy in the group will arise; hopefully this philosophy will encompass the idea that each person is worthy of respect and has the same rights as other human beings. Situations in which comfort is founded on proving someone else wrong or evading accountability for one's actions should be avoided.

Initiating feedback for change

By decreasing threats to self-esteem and increasing members' sense of security, the nurse prepares the group to be open to feedback from one another about their behavior. Of vital importance to the role of the nurse is the capacity of the group to recognize the nature of their behavior and the consequences this behavior has in terms of interactions with others. Berne, in referring to games such as wooden-leg and peasant, suggests that once behavior patterns such as these are identified by the leader and acknowledged by clients, they are subject to review, reversal, or modification. It is important that the leader initiate a process of feedback exchange between himself and the group and among members that facilitates their realization of fixed patterns of relating. First the leader must be cognizant of the fact that the behavior observed can be typed along various dimensions and in light of members' contributions to the group development or individuals' progress toward personal growth or both. Once the leader has sufficiently identified the behavior, this patterned response can be brought to the awareness of the group so that others can comment about what they have observed and what effect this behavior has had on them. It is important that the members whose behaviors are being scrutinized by the group are not severely threatened by this activity. The group must understand that acknowledging and analyzing behavior is a necessary ingredient in the learning process and that each person will at some point be given feedback about his behavior. By requiring the group to look at specific behaviors, the leader encourages them to be more sophisticated about how internal fears are manifested in actions and how these actions then stimulate reactions in others. In addition to acknowledging the nature of one's behavior, it is just as important to discuss the consequences of the behavior in terms of total interaction. It is through this discussion that the group acquires added insight into why the behavior occurs and how complex the relationships are in the group setting. The opinions and insights of the total group can be particularly helpful to the individual in that he learns the perceptions of a variety of people. If individuals gain a sound knowledge of the nature of their behavior and its effects on others, they are better equipped to decide whether they wish to maintain or modify this behavior. Since change is the norm in the group and the objective for all members, the individual is supported in his desires to experiment with new behavior patterns. These new behaviors should allow him more flexibility and more fruitful interpersonal exchange and also the opportunity to contribute more constructively in reaching the aims of the group as a whole.

The leader must remember that it is not easy for members to give up fixed patterns of relating. These patterns are learned adaptations that have served the individual's cause repeatedly. With some members it will seem almost impossible to jar him free. In my own experience with persons who achieve a great deal of secondary gain and do not really want to give up a pattern I have at times felt helpless and hopeless. In some cases I will confront a couple or individual frankly, explaining that adherence to the "Yes, but . . ." game or utilization of "wooden-leg" is getting them nowhere, and they will have to exert conscious control over these patterns.

Lastly the leader must keep in mind that when or if change does come about in some persons it can elicit anxiety on the part of the other members. This is because change in one member may produce a gap or void that the group has not counted on. For example, if a monopolizer changes his way of reacting to the group by ceasing his monopoly of group discussion, then the rest of the group will need to change and be more actively engaged in speaking in the group. What the group may or may not realize is that over a period of time it has grown to rely on the monopolizer to relieve others from having to speak to issues being discussed. The group has been able to maintain its passive silent role because it had a monopolizer. The leader's task then would be oversimplified if it were defined as simply overseeing change in individuals. The nurse must help the group recognize the complementary nature of behavior patterns and must facilitate total group movement as well as change in individual members.

REFERENCES

1. Benne, K. D., and Sheats, P.: Functional roles of group members, J. Soc. Issues **4:**41-49, 1948.
2. Berne, E.: Games people play, New York, 1964, Grove Press.
3. Berne, E.: Group treatment, New York, 1964, Grove Press.
4. Cartwright, D., and Zander, A., editors: Group dynamics, ed. 3, New York, 1968, Harper & Row, Publishers, pp. 381-387.
5. Lifton, W. M.: Working with groups, ed. 2, New York, 1967, John Wiley & Sons, p. 115.
6. Satir, V.: Conjoint family therapy, Palo Alto, Calif., 1964, Science and Behavior Books.

SUGGESTED READINGS
Group dynamics viewpoints

Bass, B., and Duntenan, G.: Behavior in groups as a function of self-interaction and task orientation, J. Abnorm. Psychol. **66:**414-428, 1963.
Bonney, W.: Pressures toward conformity in group counseling, Personnel Guidance J. **43:** 970-973, 1965.
Carter, H., and Shriver, L.: The behavior of leaders and other group members. In Cartwright, D., and Zander, A., editors: Group dynamics, ed. 3, New York, 1968, Harper & Row, Publishers, pp. 381-388.

Guetzkow, H.: The differentiation of roles in task-oriented groups. In Cartwright, D., and Zander, A., editors: Group dynamics, ed. 3, New York, 1968, Harper & Row, Publishers, pp. 512-526.

Psychotherapeutic and psychiatric viewpoints

Bateson, G.: A theory of play and fantasy, Psychiatr. Res. Rep. Am. Psychiatr. Assoc. **2:**39-51, 1955.

Berne, E.: Transactional analysis, New York, 1961, Grove Press.

Cohn, B., Ohlsen, H., and Proff, E.: Roles played by adolescents in an unproductive counseling group, Personnel Guidance J. **38:**724-731, 1960.

Jackson, D.: Interactional psychotherapy. In Stein, M., editor: Contemporary psychotherapies, Glencoe, Ill., 1962, The Free Press.

Ryckoff, I., Day, J., and Wynne, L.: Maintenance of stereotyped roles in families of schizophrenics, Arch. Gen. Psychiatry **1:**93-98, 1959.

Szasz, T.: The myth of mental illness, foundations of a theory of personal conduct, New York, 1961, Hoeber Medical Division, Harper & Row, Publishers.

Implications for leader intervention

Goulding, R.: New directions in transactional analysis: creating an environment for redecision and change. In Sager, C., and Kaplan, H., editors: Progress in group and family therapy, New York, 1972, Brunner/Mazel, pp. 105-135.

Lieberman, R.: Behavioral approaches to family and couple therapy. In Sager, C., and Kaplan, H., editors: Progress in group and family therapy, New York, 1972, Brunner/Mazel, pp. 329-346.

Loomis, M. E., and Dodenhoff, J. T.: Working with informal patient groups, Am. J. Nurs. **70:** 1939-1944, 1970.

Nikelly, A. G., editor: Techniques for behavior change, Springfield, Ill., 1971, Charles C Thomas, Publisher.

Journals

Small Group Behavior—An International Journal of Therapy, Counseling, and Training
Journal of Applied Behavior
International Journal of Group Psychotherapy

CHAPTER 13

Special techniques

Introduction

Generally derived from the world of psychotherapy, yet also drawn from the disciplines of education, art, dance, and drama, are a number of special techniques employed in groups. These techniques include games, improvisations, and exercises. They can depend heavily on theater skills and various media, such as audiovisual aids, or exist completely without them. Techniques can be extremely useful with groups whose members are not verbally articulate or whose concerns can only be arrived at through spontaneous interaction with others. In most instances techniques are adjuncts to—and *not* the essence of—the group process and group experience. They serve as the means by which the leader can accomplish goals in the group, not as ends in themselves. In general they have been known to help individuals develop insight, to encourage experimentation with new ways of behaving, and to help individuals develop understanding of other persons and the basis of behavior.

Techniques have been employed in a variety of contexts. They have been used as a medium to handle individual problems and to ease the passage through phases of trust, control, and affection. They have been used to help solve interracial problems, as well as marriage and family problems, to help individuals deal with suppressing organizations, and to supplement the vocational training of persons in small groups.

The widespread use of techniques is, however, relatively recent. The reason special techniques have found an audience in group therapy is probably a result of many factors. Group leaders, particularly in the last two decades, have found that group experiences acquire additional relevancy and have a greater practical base if groups adopt methods of learning by doing. It seemed more meaningful for some groups to role play certain interpersonal problems than to merely talk about them. Techniques have been found to be most useful in situations where the group experience was short but nevertheless had to achieve certain benefits. Some techniques, blindman's walk, for example, elicit feelings of trust in a group that may have taken some time to develop without the use of this technique. Techniques such as this are especially useful in short-term group experiences.

In addition, certain interpersonal problems of members seemed to necessitate the employment of techniques to increase the authenticity of human exchange and to promote experimentation with behaviors. As groups began to deal more and more with helping relatively well persons achieve self-actualization, the need for an action-oriented, as opposed to a purely discussion-oriented, format became apparent.

The employment of techniques requiring both action and "acting out" served to cut through intellectualizing behavior in a group as well as to promote open experimentation in dealing with others.

Chronically disabled communicators also seemed to benefit from the use of techniques. In instances where social ineptness was caused by the inability to communicate verbally with people or by a mistrust of verbal communication, "things to do" in the group provided members with an alternative mode of beginning and forming relationships with one another. Fantasy games like "What I would do if I had a million dollars . . ." would ease members into getting to know each other and into getting to members' more vital concerns.

Leaders of a patient group in a day treatment center realized they had reached a plateau in assisting members to improve on their problem-solving and social skills. Members showed disinterest in traditional talking modes of sharing problems. These patients had had many years of therapy with several kinds of group therapy approaches. The leaders decided to structure the entire group experience utilizing special techniques. They adopted a simplified encounter—sensitivity training model using self-improvement, life enrichment experiences, and weekly goal-setting exercises. Body image exercises, surveys, and telling stories were incorporated activities.

Consequently the group decreased talking about past events and focused more on relevant "here-and-now" experiences; members knew each others' names, showed concern for one another, showed pride in the group, and increased socialization activities outside the group. The overall effect then was to enhance members' movement at a time when the old and usual methods lacked potency in changing this client group.

In general, then, special techniques and those that we will describe here serve various functions. Techniques can get members involved, and in particular, involved in the exchange of feedback and feelings. Techniques also quickly get members to interact in different ways with one another. Since they can vary the type and intensity of interaction between members, they can stimulate group discussion so that further insight can occur on several levels. Also, since techniques require members to act out various situations, as opposed to merely talking about them, they can decrease the intellectualization that goes on in a group and encourage spontaneity in the group's ability to work with interpersonal concerns. Finally, techniques have a basis in simulation and re-creation of events because they can decrease the use of defenses in general and increase experimentation with new modes of relating. The nurse group leader who has a foundation of experience with basic principles and practices of group work will find the inclusion of a repertoire of special techniques a most valuable addition, lending flexibility and creativity to one's practice.

In the following discussion several techniques currently employed in group psychotherapy and therapeutic and growth groups will be isolated and described. These techniques will be categorized according to the specific outcome desired by the group leader, such as building trust, developing body awareness, releasing tension and expressing aggression, confronting conflicts and frustrations through action, and accepting positive feelings of giving and receiving positive feedback. In addition, special attention will be given to two techniques that tend to have multiple outcomes for members. These techniques are role playing and psychodrama, which are more specialized than specific outcome techniques and tend to effect various outcomes, depending on the focus of the role-playing or psychodrama experience.

Examples of techniques
Building trust

Among those techniques most widely used in groups are techniques that accelerate or otherwise enhance the establishment of trust between members. The two trust-building techniques described here are blindman's walk and the rolling (sometimes referred to as the rocking) exercise described by Schutz.[4] Both techniques focus on the issue of trust by encouraging members to put themselves in the hands of another person.

Blindman's walk requires members to divide up into pairs, sometimes with the person they trust least in the group. Each pair takes turns in leading one another around the room with one member wearing a blindfold. As one is led around the room, he must experience trusting one other person. After this exercise is completed, members discuss their feelings about trusting and being trusted. To feel completely comfortable in this situation persons must have full confidence in themselves and their partners; often this exercise causes members to confront and resolve their feelings of mistrust in one another.

The rolling exercise has basically the same effect. With persons making a circle, each individual in turn comes to the center of the circle and is passed around by the other group members. He is asked to relax as completely as possible. The discussion that follows this exercise focuses on how it felt to be passed around by virtual strangers but also on how it felt to be responsible for another's well-being.

With both blindman's walk and the rolling exercise members act out the issue of trust—whether to trust or not to trust and whether to be trustworthy. Persons confront fears of personal involvement with others, which may relate to concerns about personal harm, losing control, too much responsibility, or destructive impulses. The leader may choose to focus on the here-and-now manifestations of these fears, delve more deeply into persons' pasts, or employ techniques merely as a means of achieving further personal involvement in the group. Although it has not been substantially documented, I believe that merely participating in these exercises liberates members from their fears of personal involvement and thereby encourages growth in the relationships between individuals in the group. It is extremely important that members spend time looking at their feelings about what they did and about what went on.

Developing body awareness

Techniques directed toward developing body awareness are quite popular. Such techniques can vary from the famous nude encounters developed in the West by Paul Bindrim of Los Angeles to the less sensational sensory awareness exercises. These techniques usually attempt to illustrate one or more of the following points to members: (1) that your body (your physical stature and so on) is a reflection of your psyche or emotional self, (2) that one can do many things with his body—things that he may not yet have done, and (3) that your body, as well as your behavior, can participate in blocking or initiating human exchanges.

There are many techniques to develop body awareness. Two which I have found to be most helpful to members are the "What am I—What do I feel?" exercise and the locking-unlocking exercise described by Schutz.[4]

The "What am I?" exercise can best be implemented in a group equipped with a closed-circuit television. Members, one at a time, view themselves on the television screen. They are free to stand, sit, move around, and otherwise explore their bodies with the use of the television camera. While they are looking at themselves on the screen, they are asked to tell the group what they see in themselves. Others in the group may verify or disagree with the individual's evaluation. Since the television can preserve action, members have the benefit of replay and of seeing themselves fully in positions they may not ordinarily take in front of a mirror. Seeing their bodies projected on the television screen has the additional advantage of helping members to look at themselves more objectively and therefore of learning more about themselves. Often members remark that they saw features they were not totally aware of, features that reflected what they were feeling, and features that they could understand would repel or attract others. One member of an encounter group I led remarked that she did not realize her smile was so quick and "thin;" it was almost as if she were sneering at people and not really enjoying their company. She realized that people might feel that she was not sincere. In addition to the feedback she received from the videotape, she was able to get feedback from others in the group as to whether they noticed her smile and how they had interpreted her facial expressions.

The locking-unlocking exercise gives members further information about how their bodies participate in human interaction. This exercise can be done with members who feel especially "locked up," as Schutz[4] suggests, or with all members at the beginning of the group. (Most persons at the outset of a group experience difficulty communicating and employ some physical posture suggesting blockage of communication.) Members are directed to unlock themselves physically, to unfold, uncross, and lay open their bodies. As individuals begin to unlock themselves physically, they are made aware of the postures they have taken. These postures are frequently defensive positions—positions to cover up or otherwise keep others from penetrating them. Many acknowledge that their "hard," controlled exteriors probably served as formidable barriers to strangers in the group who wanted to get to know them. Generally the group is astonished that their new physical openness requires far less energy to maintain. Individuals report how much more comfortable they feel in talking and how less distant everyone else seems to be. Members may want to go on and experience other ways of unfolding, for example, getting up, walking around, swinging arms, or running and skipping. They realize that their locking up not only was a response to their anxiety about being in the group but also was dictated by what they thought was acceptable and expected behavior in a group setting. The group learns that they can do many things with their bodies, that persons make certain choices, and that these choices contribute to, as well as reflect, their openness in relating to others. This form of learning seems extremely useful to groups as a whole and particularly helpful to persons who have not achieved an overall sense of body awareness and a knowledge of the manifestations of nonverbal communication.

Releasing tension and expressing aggression

Aggression and hostility frequently occur in groups, for example, between marriage partners or between two members who disagree. Most of the time it is hidden or covert. It either can result from a buildup of hostilities over a long period of time and involve members' relations outside the context of the group or can arise out of the interaction in the group sessions. Frequently members have not adopted sufficient means to handle their feelings of hostility so that a great deal of tension is spent in coping with them covertly.

Several techniques or exercises can be employed to help members clarify and dissipate these feelings of hostility and aggression, as well as to help them express these feelings in a productive and acceptable way. The first two exercises described here are useful when members' feelings of aggression are due to some general source of frustration.

Slashing the air and shadowboxing are two techniques described by Schutz[4] to release tension caused by hostility or aggression. Altogether, or one at a time, members participate by striking out at an invisible opponent without fear of the energy or power that is expressed when they are flinging their arms in the air or poking their fists at their own shadow. The group that has at its disposal materials such as punching bags has the added advantage of providing members with tangible but acceptable targets. A tangible target allows members insights into what it means to hit out but also what it means to feel the hurt or pain of inflicting a blow.

Fight games are exercises that bring members in direct physical contact with one another for the purpose of expressing aggression and relieving tension. Individuals may be advised to refrain from using weapons other than themselves but are encouraged to fight with one another using a number of means, for example, pulling, pushing, or punching if these activities are suited to them. Fight games are especially helpful to couples and families with deep-seated aggressions or for persons who cannot fight openly—who fear their own power or the power of others. Two members at a time enter the center of the circle and begin fighting as the rest of the group observes to gain insight or simply to get vicarious pleasure from the combat. Usually the leader is designated as the official referee; still, members themselves employ their own inhibitions and, if anything, need encouragement from the leader to "put yourself into it."

After the exercise is completed, members discuss their methods of fighting and how they felt about what they did. Individuals frequently marvel at the fact that they could really fight and "no one got hurt that much." Sometimes members remark that they feel much closer to their sparring partner and that their feelings of hostility were not clear cut—that they may have felt jealousy, admiration, and even some af-

fection toward the other person. It is extremely useful for observers, as well as participants, to talk about what happened and how they felt. Observers may express that
they felt protective toward one of the fighters, felt the sparring partners were faking,
or felt frustrated that they could not join in. Talking about how they felt during the
"fight" will give them further opportunity to release their own tensions, as well as
make them aware of their own feelings about physical combat or overt expressions of
aggression. Fight games can help the entire group arrive at a new level of ease just
by allowing members to ventilate the tension they have built up through physical
combat.

Confronting conflicts and frustrations through action

Closely related to fight games are a number of exercises designed for members
to confront various conflicts through action. In any group situation persons experience certain conflicts or frustrations associated with belonging to a group and meeting the expectations of group membership. One of the most common issues around
group membership with which every member must come to terms is whether he truly wants to be "in" or "out." Frustrations around the issue of in or out may become
more acute when members sense impending isolation or alienation from the group
or when they feel enveloped by group standards and norms.

Breaking-in and breaking-out exercises, described by Schutz[4] and the Human
Development Institute[1] help members confront this conflict directly. At the beginning of either exercise the leader relates the activities to the personal issue of affiliation with the group. To complete the breaking-out exercise, individuals are asked to
stand in a circle and, one at a time, step outside. Outside the circle persons are encouraged to break in, using whatever means they can. In essence, members are
asked to experience the frustrations of trying to be a part of the "in group," while
others try hard to keep the person from breaking in.

Quite the opposite of the breaking-in exercise is the breaking-out technique.
Breaking out brings the frustrations of members about being too involved and too
controlled by the group to surface. Individuals experience on the one hand the pleasure of definitive boundaries and on the other hand the misery of being confined, de-
layed, or restricted. With persons standing in a circle, each member is asked to go to
the center and then is instructed to face the frustration of being enveloped by the
group and to actively participate in breaking loose by breaking out of the circle. To
their dismay others will do everything they can to keep them inside. When individuals do finally physically break through and discharge their frustrations about being
locked in, they are met with sudden freedom from boundaries. This sense of freedom
can make them realize that neither being pinned in nor being completely out is what
they desire. The group is encouraged to talk about this conflict and what alternatives
there are in terms of involvement in the group. This discussion frequently leads to
examining a much broader issue dealing with how one can preserve his integrity
and still accommodate the requisites of group membership.

It is important to note here that the breaking-out exercise, like many of the other
participative exercises or techniques, can be used for more than one purpose. The

Human Development Institute encounter tapes use breaking out to help members identify and compare the different ways that people cope with the same problem. Each member is asked to take his turn in breaking out of the circle. Group members discuss the various tactics used in dealing with the common problem of breaking out. The frustration members face here is basically the same; the discussion, however, deals with how individuals solve the same problem. Although the activity is the same, the focus of the discussion changes and therefore makes the objective of the exercise somewhat different. One point needs further emphasis here; that is, it is not the exercise itself which in the last analysis determines what members will learn. Rather it is how the leader defines and describes the task and in what direction he guides the discussion following the exercise that is most crucial to the outcome.

Accepting positive feelings: giving and receiving

It is not unusual for people to experience difficulty in giving or receiving positive feedback, or in both. In part this is a problem of simply not being able to feel "good" about another person, but it is also a problem in believing that oneself can be loved, admired, respected, or adored. Persons may have difficulty in accepting positive feedback as genuine. They may not hear positive feedback from others, or they may only believe negative feedback.

Give and take (or giving and receiving, as designed by Schutz) and strength bombardment (designed by Herbert Otto) are two exercises that relate to these problems of self-esteem. Strength bombardment requires members to focus only on their "good" points and to receive positive feedback from the group. Each person tells the rest of the group about his good points or strengths and then listens to what the group says are his attributes. The opportunity to focus only on one's strengths tends to promote a feeling of increased self-esteem. In addition, however, persons experience the difficulties they have either in receiving positive feedback or in giving it to another. The elation that follows this experience can be mixed with puzzlement. Members wonder why they were uncomfortable in hearing good things about themselves or why it was hard to think of good things to say about other persons in the group. The fact that some members can only accept negative appraisals is usually enlightening to the total group. On the whole, however, this experience is more affective than productive of any profound intellectual insights. It may not be until later sessions that the full impact of persons' ability to give and receive takes on intellectual meaning.

Give and take can either substitute for strength bombardment or can build on what was accomplished by this latter exercise. With strength bombardment, also, persons experience themselves as valued, thus adding to their self-esteem. Give and take can also add the dimension of nonverbal expression of feelings. Members are told to select others from the group who they think have trouble letting people get close to them. One at a time the selected individuals enter the circle. Other group members take turns approaching the person in the center and nonverbally or verbally expressing the positive feelings they have toward him. This exercise is also effective if the person in the center is advised to receive this expression without returning it. He has the full effect of receiving without being obligated to give back. The discussion that follows this exercise can focus on many fruitful issues: (1) how one can convey feelings through nonverbal expressions if nonverbal expression was made a part of the exercise, (2) what persons felt comfortable in doing to show their feelings, and (3) what forms of contact were avoided (such as, handshaking seemed easy, but hugging was not). With this exercise it is important for members to express how it felt to receive positive feedback and not be able to return it.

Techniques with multiple outcomes: role playing and psychodrama

Before proceeding to discuss certain points about the implementation of any technique in a group, it is important to mention two additional techniques that are basic in the operation of many groups for the purposes of occupational training or psychotherapy in the group setting. These techniques are role playing and psychodrama. Rather than explore these techniques in detail here, and indeed there are entire books written solely about these techniques, we will describe and compare the two, highlighting their essential features.

As opposed to specific outcome techniques, role playing and psychodrama are usually employed continuously throughout the group as a mode of group problem solving. Depending on their particular focus, they can achieve a variety of outcomes with a number of problems. They can focus upon the here-and-now interaction of the group or they can deal with problems of individual members that are external to the life of the group. Both role playing and psychodrama allow persons to act out interpersonal situations rather than just verbalize them.

Moreno and his co-workers, the founders of psychodrama, developed a number of methods appropriate for stimulating awareness and releasing tensions of members in a group.[3] Basic to psychodrama is (1) the presence of an alter ego and (2) role reversal. One or more members act out situations while alter egos stand beside them and indicate what these players may be feeling or thinking. Alter egos are responsible for bringing into the open true feelings or thoughts and thereby creating insight into interpersonal interaction. Members are encouraged to replay actual situations so that they can achieve some sense of mastery over what had caused them personal distress in the original situation. They are also encouraged to change roles so that they get an idea of the situations of other actors in the incident—to put themselves in the shoes of the other person so that they get a better understanding of the dynamics of human interchange.

Somewhat like psychodrama, role playing also stimulates insight into interpersonal relationships through simulation of events. Whereas alter ego functions or roles are not a part of role playing, the reversal of roles is quite frequently employed to increase individuals' understanding of other people and of behavior in general. Essentially, several members of the group replay an interpersonal problem situation, taking on various roles of the original participants. Frequently the person who originally participated in the event is encouraged to take the role of another actor before playing his own part once again. When members reenact a situation, they must guess what others were thinking, feeling, or trying to convey. The group gets a better perception of the complexity of communication and develops increased sensitivity to their own and others' behavior.

The unreal or staged aspect of role playing can be avoided if members can simulate a problem that they have had inside the group. They can face a problem of their own in the group, for example, an issue around the development of the group, and role play the possible solutions suggested by various persons. Essentially the group uses these role-playing sessions as a laboratory where they can test solutions to interpersonal problems right in the group meetings.

Role playing in particular has been used for a variety of educational purposes, most common of which is the development of interpersonal relationship skills. It is quite useful in promoting mastery over interpersonal situations for management. And, as Klein[2] suggests, one particular benefit that seems to be well documented is its ability to enhance the interpersonal functioning of persons. With role playing, as with psychodrama, members can risk learning, they can observe and analyze more objectively because the situation is a simulated one. Especially with role playing where members must feel free to make mistakes and learn by these mistakes, the element of simulation is extremely important. It can eliminate certain tensions that generate when a situation is real and therefore charged with emotion and fears. In role playing it is important that the personal, subjective element be removed sufficiently so that members experiment with new ways of behaving and increase their understanding of a situation, but not so much that the exercise loses meaning and relevancy for the group.

It is important here to point out the various assumptions that underlie role playing and psychodrama: (1) simulated situations can retain enough realism that meaningful learning can occur, and (2) if a person replays a situation, when he faces that same situation a third time, outside the group, he will employ certain skills he acquired through the replay exercise. With role playing in particular it is felt that the person who takes the role again in the real world, where it counts, *becomes* the part and is able to function effectively with the new frame of reference he acquired from his participation in the role-playing exercise.

Employing techniques and the role of the nurse leader

In planning for the best execution of techniques in the group the leader needs to take into account certain basic structural features of the group, that is, the size and duration of the group, the physical arrangements in the meeting place, and characteristics of participants. For the best use of techniques it is wise to keep the size of the group small, to approximately eight to ten persons, and to allow at least 90 minutes per group session. One must keep in mind that any technique requires time— time to describe the exercise, time to actually complete the activity, and sufficient time for summary and discussion. In some instances, time to replay the exercise is also important.

Since techniques require physical movement and sometimes much bodily activity, it is necessary to meet in a room large enough to permit movement and equipped with movable furniture. It is helpful if the room is well ventilated and yet sufficiently private to absorb noise and prevent persons from feeling overly self-conscious.

In selecting group members to participate in the various exercises the leader should keep two important points in mind. Persons who volunteer will be more motivated to learn from these experiences, and exercises that require deep emotional involvement would best be done with persons who demonstrate emotional stability and function reasonably well in their day-to-day lives.

The leader should always keep in mind that techniques for the most part are advanced means of achieving certain ends in the group. It is clear then that their execution should be given much thought, that all members may not benefit by participating, and that the leader should have certain basic skills and knowledges before attempting to use them in a group.

In some groups where techniques or exercises are the total program of the group, a professional trainer or leader may not be necessary, but usually the group is directed in some way by skillfully trained persons. An example of such a situation is the encountertapes used by the Western Behavioral Science Institute, which direct a group's activity through a planned program relayed by a moderator on the tapes.

I believe that for any leader to employ techniques effectively he must possess a great deal of knowledge and skill. For example, the leader must be able to recognize key interpersonal concerns manifested in groups, as well as when they are likely to occur and what types of issues or problems are best dealt with in other than a discussion manner. Group leaders must be able to stimulate group members to abandon previous means of handling problems, for example, through intellectualization, in order to bring them to an action-oriented way of working with them. They must know not only how to direct an exercise or technique but also how to utilize the action and outcome of the activity in a fruitful discussion so that members develop increased insight and acquire added personal growth. The selection and utilization of techniques should be based on sound theoretical knowledge, an adequate assessment of the problems of members, the purposes of techniques, and the meaning of personal growth for individuals. In essence, to execute the role of leader one must be fully prepared to plan and design the action, direct the procedures, and develop the sequence of events in a thoroughly meaningful way for persons with a variety of needs and strengths. The minimal requisites as I view them are (1) experience and study in groups to know when and how typical problems are manifested in a group setting, (2) an understanding of interpersonal and communication problems of individuals at various stages of wellness or illness, and (3) a beginning orientation to techniques including demonstrations of how they may be employed in a variety of situations.

Inside the group even the most experienced group leader needs to check and recheck the use of techniques. Conscientiousness must at the same time be mediated by a certain spontaneity and eagerness for members to discover and learn with these tools.

Basic to success with exercises in the group, however, are several aspects of administration worth noting and emphasizing. Time and timing is extremely important. Cramming too many techniques into one session is a common pitfall. Members become overloaded with stimuli and have difficulty sorting out their feelings and insights. It is far better to utilize one technique in depth than to require members to run through exercises in drill fashion.

This brings us to still another point about timing. Each exercise or technique requires a certain amount of time not only to complete an exercise but also to discuss it and perhaps to replay the interaction until the group is satisfied. With role playing in particular one interactional problem may be replayed two or three times before the group is totally satisfied with the outcome. Each replay, although it focuses on aspects of the same problem, may bring up different feelings and new insights that should be discussed. Briefly there are no shortcuts; once an exercise is begun, time should be allotted for every phase of its development.

Another problem with the use of exercises frequently encountered by group leaders is that of overprogramming the group. Overprogramming as to what is expected through the use of a tool has the effect of restricting members' experience to a certain set of outcomes. Members are not free to experience the exercise in new ways that are unique to their own needs and personalities. Overprogramming usually occurs when the leader is overzealous in describing the technique and projects onto the current group the desire that they profit from what other groups have experienced.

I personally have confronted this situation with supervisees who have been through a recent self-actualization group experience and wish to impose, without alteration, all those techniques that were used on them. Still enchanted by their own experience, they do not realize that they may be expecting unrealistic outcomes for patients or clients with different levels of wellness than was true for themselves. This does not mean, however, that the leader should not define and describe what activities are expected of the group members in order to complete the exercise. In giving this description, however, the leader should be mindful of the problem of overprogramming the group as to what should occur.

Along this same line leaders should gear their own participation so that members can sufficiently express themselves and experience the exercise without constant interruption. Intervening with too much description or with too many observations and interpretations can have the same effect as overprogramming. That is, members are not given sufficient opportunity to participate in ways that are meaningful to them.

The leader must always be cognizant of discomfort members feel when they are asked to participate in exercises. Simulation and acting out feelings and frustrations are foreign to many people. For the most part individuals may use other means to cope with situations that the leader is now asking them to handle through action. Members may voice their difficulties in "getting in the mood," their uneasiness and feeling "on the spot," or generally feeling silly, self-conscious, or embarrassed. Some of these feelings are transient and disappear with completion of one or more exercises. Members begin to see the value in the exercise or begin to get wrapped up in what they are doing and what they are learning to the extent that they have forgotten to be concerned with how they appear. Still, in all this, the leader should avoid placing anyone on the spot who does not feel support from the group. Being put on the spot without sympathy and understanding from others is unusually cruel and is undeserving punishment unless it is the task of members to master these very feelings. As the leader gets more and more experience with the use of techniques, it will become easier for him to discern those exercises that tend to make people feel uncomfortable and those individuals who feel more vulnerable than others. It then becomes the task of the leader to take the pressure off by whatever means is appropriate at the time. It is important before starting emotion-ladened exercises that the leader explain that anyone who does not feel like participating has the option of "sitting it out" as long as he remains in the group to observe what goes on.

Avoiding putting members on the spot brings up two additional points every leader should be aware of. First is that the leader should know and take into account the feelings, fears, and desires that may be aroused by a particular technique. The leader must be equipped to help persons deal with these reactions when they occur. Too often leaders become so wrapped up in the here-and-now activity of the exercise that they lose track of what is happening with persons in the group. Near the close of the session as group members' concerns become more evident, there may not be enough time to deal with them adequately. If the leader was cognizant of the particular result of a technique and kept this in mind, the reactions may have been anticipated and planned for more judiciously.

Second, no technique or exercise should be attempted unless the group and the leader understand how to use it and the leader feels sure that it is appropriate. With the recent trend in the use of techniques and their reported positive impact on persons, some leaders have gone full-steam ahead and adopted action-oriented tools without having a sufficient understanding of how they should be used. Necessarily they cannot adequately explain the use of the exercises to the group, and the exercises' potential benefits are not realized. At this point the discouraged leader may disclaim their usefulness and avoid gaining additional knowledge and skill in their use. To the extent that these tools are new and, in essence, current fads, the probability of their misuse or abuse is great. The need for evaluating the effect of special techniques is clear. Much more research should be directed at documenting the relative impact of these experiential exercises. The leader should keep in mind that there is no excuse for employing interventions of any kind without some knowledge of how these interventions should be employed and of what results are to be expected.

One last and final point that every leader should keep in mind when utilizing techniques in groups is that these techniques are the *means*, not the ends, of the total group experience. Unlike more subtle interventions, these tools are dramatic and time consuming and may be mistaken for the ends instead of the means. Members, as well as the leader, may forget that there was some underlying reason for engaging in their activities. If the leader keeps in mind the purpose of the exercise, the group is more likely to be guided toward this purpose, utilizing their involvement in the exercise to instruct them in an area where learning needs to occur. The leader not only should state the purpose of the activity at the outset but also should summarize the experience in light of this objective.

To do justice to this area of group specialization and to the role of the nurse group leader, we need to end on a more positive note. The use of techniques and exercises is rising in popularity. Understandably so, for these tools present an exciting and dynamic approach to looking at human problems in the context of a group setting. For persons who have difficulty in verbally articulating their interpersonal concerns and who are prompted by simulated circumstances and for those who learn better when understanding is arrived at through spontaneous interaction with others, these action-oriented exercises present an important supplement to group work. The advanced nurse group leader whose skills and interests lie in the area of creative involvement with individuals will find techniques to be the freshest approach to group work known to leaders today.

REFERENCES
1. Human Development Institute: Encountertapes for personal growth groups, La Jolla, Calif., 1968, Western Behavioral Sciences Institute.
2. Klein, A. F.: Role playing in leadership training and group problem solving, New York, 1961, Association Press.
3. Moreno, J. L.: Psychodrama, New York, 1946, Beacon House.
4. Schutz, W.: Joy-expanding human awareness, New York, 1967, Grove Press.

SUGGESTED READINGS
Berzon, B., and Solomon, L. N.: The self-directed group: a new direction in personal growth learning. In Hart, J. T., and Tomlinson, T. M., editors: New directions in client-centered psychotherapy, Boston, 1968, Houghton Mifflin Co.
Bradshaw, J.: Techniques used in sensitivity training. Unpublished essay.
Brooks, D.: Teletherapy: or how to use videotape feedback to enhance group process, Perspect. Psychiatr. Care **14:**83-87, 1976.
Burton, N.: Videotape playback as a therapeutic device in group psychotherapy, Int. J. Group Psychother. **19:**433-440, 1969.
Dodge, C.: A review of the use of audiovisual equipment in psychotherapy, Perspect. Psychiatr. Care **7:**248-257, 1969.
Hogan, P., and Alger, I.: The impact of videotape recording on insight in group psychotherapy, Int. J. Group Psychother. **19:**158-164, 1969.
Howard, J.: Please touch, New York, 1970, McGraw-Hill Book Co.
Johnson, D., and Johnson, F.: Joining together—group theory and group skills, Englewood Cliffs, N.J., 1975, Prentice-Hall.
Johnson, D.: Role reversal: a summary and review of the research, Int. J. Group Tensions **1:**318-334, 1971.
Kaseman, B.: An experimental use of structured techniques in group psychotherapy, Group Psychother. Psychodrama Sociometry **29:**33-39, 1976.
Leiberman, M., Yalom, I., and Miles, M.: Encounter groups, first frets, New York, 1973, Basic Books, Inc., Publishers.
Levitsky, A., and Perls, F.: The rules and games of Gestalt therapy, San Francisco, 1976, San Francisco Gestalt Therapy Institute. Available from the Institute, 3701 Sacramento St., San Francisco, Calif.
Rogers, C. R.: The process of the basic encounter group. In Bugental, J. F. T., editor: Challenge of humanistic psychology, New York, 1967, McGraw-Hill Book Co.
Schein, E., and Bennis, W. G.: Personal and organizational change through group methods, New York, 1965, John Wiley & Sons.

Schiffman, M.: Self-therapy techniques for personal growth, Menlo Park, Calif., 1971, Self Therapy Press.

Stoller, F.: Focused feedback with videotape: extending the group's functions. In Gazda, G., editor: Basic innovations in group psychotherapy and counseling, Springfield, Ill., 1969, Charles C Thomas, Publisher.

Zweben, J., and Hammann, S.: Prescribed games: a theoretical perspective on the use of group techniques, Psychother. Theory Res. Pract. **7:**22-27, 1970.

Index